The Power of Mental Toughness

Techniques for Peak Athletic Performance

High3r Mindset

"You don't get handed mental toughness, you have to grow it."

ISBN: 978-1-7387390-2-8

The Power of Mental Toughness

Table of Contents

Introduction

More than ever before, more and more people identify as athletes. The amount and quality of information regarding performance and training available now far surpass what has been thought possible a generation ago, with many amateurs now accessing and using information that was not long ago reserved only for national-level sportspeople.

The common use of wearable technology combined with online platforms lets us compare our performances globally, along with the vast array of methods and factors influencing results that have exploded and syncretized what were once competing for methodologies. This body of data is truly incredible, with a massive amount of meta-data that lets us instantly correlate any element we want. Smart use of coaches and data collection lets us analyze what we do in a way that is changing sports performance fundamentally, in part by exposing old myths and identifying the fundamentals of performance that are key to all sports as real determining factors of success.

Emerging rapidly as a primary element of performance is the concept of Mental Toughness, something you will have probably seen mentioned everywhere from serious research to advertising on supplements. This term is often only vaguely defined at best, relying more on the emotional impact of the sound and allusions, and though we all know what it means at an intuitive level, in the world of athletic conversation, not much is clear.

Once a vague notion more associated with only endurance athletics or sports like mountaineering, mental toughness is being shown to be part of the basis of performance common to all sports, as the attributes that it includes are seen to influence performance. Where once it was noticed only as a factor in competition, we now know that mental toughness is also the basis for preparation and training.

The Toughened Mind

Mental toughness is a cumbersome term, but it leaves little question as to what it infers and is literally what it 'says on the tin'. Other terms, such as *resilience* and *fortitude* of course exist to label the same thing but require a degree of explanation that can leave out nuance and details.

The attribute of mental toughness simply means having a mind toughened against pressures that can undermine it. This infers a mind that has been strengthened and trained to be better controlled under pressure and less swayed by outside forces because it has been instilled with the attributes that the usual factors for stress cannot affect.

The toughened mind becomes proofed against all the things that detract from our abilities, which include anxiety, fatigue, distraction, corruption, small-mindedness, impatience, distorted identity, impatience, and undeveloped attitudes toward the process of competition. In the context of athleticism, these things can act like dominoes when under pressure, so that when one attribute is weak, it influences the others to cause a chain reaction where the athlete cannot come back.

Tough also mean being structurally robust, not just simply calloused to stress and distraction. Being mentally tough is not to be so basic as to have no finer faculties that could be weaknesses, but to have developed all faculties so they can stand up to the rigors of performance, competition, and extended training. Without a structure for the mind's traits to be organized, even the finest attributes cannot be put effectively towards purpose, and in athleticism, that purpose is the cauldron of competition.

Combined, the faculties of mental toughness form what is called the athlete's character, something they will be judged by in every aspect, not just in how they compete. This character is what the athlete presents to the world as well as being the thing they navigate the world by, and a well-developed character that is mentally tough makes an impressive presence when it comes time to perform.

Getting Some

We all know people that are mentally tough, but not all people who are mentally tough know that they are. Usually, the first sign of true mental toughness is a reluctance to assign the label to themselves, because the very attributes of perspective, self-validation, and gratitude, among others, reject the notion that what they are is so easily confirmed.

No one is born mentally tough, but for many, it is something they develop by circumstance in their formative years. Athletes that come from backgrounds that have seen great pressure or change will often have some of the traits of mental toughness they have needed to rely on throughout their lives. This may mean difficult life circumstances or simply growing up in an environment of hard work, where things like climate and work choices demand a lot of their character.

Other athletes will have developed toughness through the effort to correct bad choices, something commonly found when the lives of great athletes are looked into. Many people with natural inclinations toward dynamic and high-risk activities, will go through several versions of tough life choices before finding athleticism as the best choice. These other choices can include all sorts of waywardness, from drugs and bad social choices to taking jobs that incur injury. The impetus is often for the commitment and excitement that these choices bring, and the lessons learned—often the hard way—transfer to athleticism well and offer a more positive future.

For the rest of us, mental toughness is something we develop through our choices, intentionally and as a product of other things we decide to do with our lives. In athletics, mental toughness is given high priority because it is what allows athletes to train and compete and developing it in this way can result in high-level performance.

Especially for the athlete that learns to acknowledge mental toughness early in their sports career, this process of development can take them to profound levels of performance. These are not traits developed quickly, and though the effects may be felt soon, the full outcomes of mental toughness accumulate over time.

The sort of mental toughness that results in elite performance comes together by being infused into every aspect of an athlete's efforts, from the choices they make in competition to the many, many hours of training. The athlete gradually develops their mind along with their abilities, with mental toughness being the thing by which they navigate their choices. The toughened mind chooses better options when it comes to preparation and performance because its faculties are better developed to be stronger and more integrated. The toughened mind has greater perspective, control, and patience to see through the long timelines that elite performance requires, gaining an advantage over others less tolerant of the workload.

As a central faculty, mental toughness is what connects the beginner athlete to the competitor that prevails months or years later at the top of their game. As an equation of time to effort, it is the best attribute to develop because it references every other aspect of the athlete's character so they can perform as a whole.

Chapter 1: Focus

Focus is the part of mental toughness that brings you the precision of thought, intent, and attention that lets you cut through all the stuff that would be vulnerabilities if you let it take up more of your mindset. This is what makes you confident, committed, and engaged, and what lets you play with the intensity dial that gets difficult stuff done.

Every mental trait, whatever it is, requires focus to develop. Focus is the mind directing itself towards a result while simultaneously blocking out anything that detracts from it. Focus also has a large physical component—reinforcing the mind-body continuum that all sports performance is built on—where the focusing of fine motor activity and bulk mass is where mental toughness becomes expressed when it is time to perform.

Focus is a very trainable faculty with an accepted and well-known range of techniques for developing it as a part of the everyday ability. Ranging from the basic and pragmatic to the bizarre and convoluted, methods for training the mind to be more focused accompany most sports and training methodologies, from the centuries-old Zen practices of Japanese martial arts to the use of flotation tanks and virtual reality.

Most of these techniques aim at conditioning the mind to respond to stimuli that the athlete uses to quiet distraction and focus attention on subtle things like the breath, mental concepts, or their reactions to things like invasive ideas or stress. Repetition and refinement gradually 'hardwire' the mind to use these principles reflexively, with the idea being that under the stress of competition and performance, the athlete will automatically slip into this trained state of focus.

Effects from even a short period of developing focus can be seen quickly in performance. Much of the efficacy is due to the way most athletes' minds will respond well to any method that increases performance. Positive contributions to mental toughness will soon be seen in the way the mind can focus more clearly and for longer. Practice creates a learning loop where the athlete's mind is developing itself based on its own increased ability; practice increases focus, focus increases practice, and so on in a cycle that makes the mind ever more able to sharpen and avoid distraction.

Meditation

The process of training the mind to focus has been recognized and practiced for thousands of years as a fundamental human skill. Our species has always known that the mind benefits from training itself to think with more precision and more intent, and doing this with meditation is something most societies understand.

Forget everything you may have thought about meditation as some kind of devotional or occult practice, because separate from all that, meditation is backed up by cold, hard science. There is no placebo here; sitting without distraction and intently bringing your thought processes to a state of focus on a single thing and intimately perceiving it from all available angles has been shown to wire in mental ability that is felt during the performance.

This especially applies to complex and systemic abilities, where weak links threaten entire sequences, which can be focused on and magnified with meditation to discern and analyze problems and solutions. Meditation's capacity as a learning tool is that increased focus lets the athlete observe further into the details of their performance, both in the meditative state and during practice and competition, and discern weaknesses and solutions. This enhanced capacity to perceive their own machinations is a powerful training tool that no external coaching or training method can provide, and is key to setting the athlete on the sort of non-generic course where unique performance is forged.

This highly informed addition to athletic preparation requires a mind ready to accept the challenges of more specialized training because this is not the world of 20-minute training sessions offered by the commercial pop-athletics media. Training like this, and the performance benefits that result, need a degree of self-confidence and mental toughness for the athlete to work with.

Focus plays out in mental toughness as both the ability to enhance the resilience of your mind's structure and a laser-like capacity to see into sports performance and do it better. Meditation here is only the method for developing these abilities, and like all methods, should not be mistaken for the goal itself. It is easy to become enamored with meditation, as it is with any training method, which requires fixation on the technique, and it is here that mental toughness is needed to keep the mental attributes aligned.

Like at the gym or track, it is important to analyze the practice of meditation to see that it is continuing to develop the mind's ability to focus. Like other aspects of training, meditation needs to come in cycles and phases, that work on various elements of focus and mental acuity.

Trained well, the focused mind stays on track longer and better, perceives weaknesses earlier, analyzes choices with greater fidelity, and remains beyond distraction with a greater bandwidth of detail. These things alone make up for a large part of toughness and are easily observed during events where toughness is what matters.

Conditioning

There is no real gap between a focused mind and focused actions, and that connection is made with conditioning.

Proper training is much more than simply preparing the body for the effort of sport, it is the honing of the fine motor skills, intentional reactions, and integrated movements so the body can focus on what the mind directs it to do. Whether it's pitching, running, a swimmer's stroke, or a climber's pull, how precise their movements are is the product of quality conditioning.

This combined conditioning of mental and physical focus is the key to an athlete pushing beyond the limits of their normal experience because it is where the potential they have is harnessed to a specific result. The years and months of continuous practice, training, and preparation that create potential are put into shape and aligned with their goal with all of the factors conditioned so that potential can be expressed. Good conditioning will have developed the various strengths, movements, and sequences to a level ready for performance so that the focus of the mind can orchestrate it all right when it matters.

Smart conditioning is a multi-faceted thing that can be a lot different from the simplistic routines many people follow in the hope they will lead to a performance edge. To address mental toughness, conditioning needs to be specific to the sport and the athlete, as well as to the environment, timeline, and group. Mental toughness needs to be addressed in all of these aspects, otherwise, you will see the common outcome of otherwise excellent athletes who are let down on the day because they were overwhelmed by an outlying factor.

Contrary to the claims of the convenient programs that flood the internet, serious conditioning does not come in generic forms that happily fit a small selection of body types. Yes, it may be correct that a very general level of conditioning will work for anyone new to athletic pursuits, where the primary goal is to simply set the person up for a regular activity, but once they can cope with the volume of training, things need to be more relevant to the sport they have chosen.

Good conditioning is a process of getting the volume of training specific to your sport that will give you a performance edge. Each sport will have its own ideal volume, and how long that volume needs to be maintained in order to have full effect. To rise above mediocrity, most sports require consistent dedication, and this is where mental toughness starts to become more and more important in determining the better athlete. Simply put; the athlete who can tolerate the most quality has the greatest chance of prevailing.

Now, 'conditioning' doesn't just mean going hard at the gym or the track. At its absolute core, conditioning means doing the correct thing—of which going hard is one element—and knowing what that is, is a mental game. To see through the weeks, months, and years of competitive conditioning takes a mind that can keep up with the constant assessing, analyzing, adjusting, and recovering it takes, which is guaranteed to include times of boredom, confusion, pain, frustration, and even fear. Even the most common and straightforward of sports such as running or soccer, when analyzed for the competition become complex and nuanced and far from something where good performance can happen with casual effort.

The toughened mind directs conditioning, so the process is both stimulating and brings results by being up for the challenges that come with pushing the body further. A clear and focused mind with a broad perspective is not distracted by the constant carousel of fad methods and supplements and will cope with the mass of data that needs consideration for better performance. Where an easily-distracted and unpredictable mind will waste energy on apparent shortcuts and tiny improvements from exotic ideas in an attempt to avoid the hard work and volume that is the reality of any training, the mind that is tough will have the patience and focus to just do what is required.

This focus is what allows the mind to keep the goal central to all the methods and programs that make up conditioning, constantly tweaking things back to the objective, so progress keeps direction. Without focus, it is easy for conditioning to go off track and become about what feels like fun rather than what is needed, wasting precious hours that become days and sabotaging the result. Programmed right and carried off with a mindset that is up to the rigor, conditioning can produce stunning results from the field to the mountain and pool. Well-conditioned athletes minimize injury and randomness that wastes time and each year or season build on their game to make life work in their sport even at an amateur level.

Chapter 2: Perspective

Perspective is the ingredient in mental toughness that lets you know what you are being mentally tough about. With a developed perspective, you know how things interconnect and how to allocate your energy to the best effect to efficiently get through the hard stuff. Without perspective, you don't even really know what the game is, let alone how to best approach it.

Without perspective, toughness is just an illusion. You can be determined and hard as nails in one respect, but when other aspects of your character are undeveloped weaknesses, you will have big gaps in your armor, and the old adage of only being as strong as your weakest link will ring true.

Perspective is the way you arrange the information you have and build the reality you are working with. Perception is *not* reality, merely a way of looking at it, and therein lies the beauty of the mind. By developing your mental faculties, you develop the world that you perceive, and can change the entire experience of sports performance.

The perspective of a toughened mind is very different from that of a mind that is compromised by distraction and anxiety. By being less influenced by unintentional factors, the toughened mind dedicates more of the athlete's energy and responses to things directly in line with their athletic objectives. This builds a bigger perspective on performance, where more details and angles are considered, and more information is known and arranged in useable ways.

Athletes with larger perspectives simply have more data to work with and position themselves within a larger field of knowledge. This can be seen with many athletes at the top of their game, where they are drawing ideas and influences from fields even way beyond their own sport, and applying them to resolve things that become integral to success. These expansive perspectives see these athletes finding training, diet, strategic, material, and data analysis methods used elsewhere, in places not considered by their competitors, that they can use to increase performance.

The Big Picture

We all know not to 'lose sight of the bigger picture, but we don't always get what the bigger picture really is and how big it can actually be. It is not uncommon to see athletes underestimate the big picture, especially when they choose to take their sport to another level, as the shift from where they are to where they are going can mean whole new magnitudes of performance.

The "big picture" is a convenient name for the greatest sum of all that affects what you are doing. This, of course, includes the sport or competition you are pursuing, but also the way it fits into everything else. The big picture includes what led up to this point, where the outcome will go, and factors like family, work, age, changes in the competition, and everyone else that intersects with you.

In its simplest form, the big picture is the world you and your sport are within, but a perspective this simplistic leaves out a lot of detail and makes things appear random that may actually be foreseeable. For your perspective to be realistic, it must take account of a multitude of details and layers, so you can make plans that will survive the tests of time and make predictions of how things will play out.

The big picture relates to mental toughness because it shows you what you are up against. This is much more than just the scale of what you are doing, but also all the complexity, depth, potential, and influences of everything involved, and these are things that are greatly enhanced with a mind that is resilient and robust.

A tough mind allows you to confront complexity, address the unknowns, and do the hard work of committing to a plan with a large scope. Athletes that punch above their weight and compete at levels that demand a lot of them have trained their mental toughness so they can handle as big a perspective as possible.

At a big picture-level athleticism looks very different from what it does as a parochial or small-minded one, and can appear confronting or intimidating to those without the mental toughness to approach it. We have all been awed by the training loads, the scope of ideas, commitment to possibility, and the intensity of athletes at levels higher than ourselves because they have perspectives and worldviews bigger than our own. Often the question gets asked about how these top athletes arrive at these levels, and always the answer includes mental toughness and the drive to prevail.

Clarity

Perspective needs clarity, otherwise, it is volatile and lacks the definition to rely on. Clarity is what allows the details of your perspective to be seen distinctly and precisely, which means they can be better understood, implemented, and communicated.

We all value clarity, and expect it from others, especially in the precise realm of athletic performance that boils things down to statistics and nuance. By developing this in ourselves, we enhance the way we look at our own abilities and all of the elements that make us perform how we do. More clarity means we get to know ourselves better, less confused by the opinions and influence of others, and from this, we build a profile of what our unique capacity can achieve.

Clarity is central to athletic performance because it means we know our objectives better and can relate to them more effectively. With clarity, we see past the veneers of expectations and prejudices and look closer at ourselves and our competitors to judge what good performance will take. Beyond the casual level of sport where the objective is simply fun, getting performance results requires a clear understanding and perspective of what is involved. As performance increases and the previously small factors around ability gain importance, this understanding becomes ever more integral to how an athlete progresses.

Clarity relates to mental toughness by letting us know what we are being tough about. Many athletes, especially early in their careers, concern themselves too much with things that have only limited importance. This is the folly of all new sports, but the sooner the athlete moves beyond it and comes to understand the core of their performance, the sooner they can settle into preparation that has a real effect. Mental toughness is the faculty used here, to step away from the wanderlust of novelty and shift the mind into the things that generate real progress. Clarity is what is needed to guide this process, so the athlete can address the details that no coach or partner can help with.

Perception

The capacity to understand what you are dealing with is perception and is the factor that puts the context into what you are trying to achieve. Perception is where the athlete's focus, clarity, and mindset are put into motion as the functional ability to perceive.

It is one thing to see and understand what is presented to you, but another thing to drive the mind into places where it must think for itself. This is where perception matters, as does the ability to navigate with the mind, and is where you will find all those things no one else can tell you.

Perceptive athletes simply see into things further than those who have not developed the ability, letting them look past the superficial appearance of things like training and standards, and deep into the core of what is really happening. This perception is partly about the focus and clarity to see what something really is, combined with the toughness and presence of mind to cope with the rigor of pulling ideas apart.

Perception is an immensely valuable attribute because it lets the athlete see more than what is apparent. To be limited by only the immediate presentation of a sport and its performance is to not see the things that serious competition is made up of, therefore closing off the mind to the aspects of progress. The perceptive player sees more into the strategy and probability of a team, the perceptive runner sees more about the effects of time on the body, and the perceptive climber knows there is more to it than just following the route.

The athlete who develops their perception takes themselves to a higher level within the sport simply because they realize more is going on, both within themselves and within the competition. They can better fill the position they have in the sport, being able to see new avenues for improvement, the advantages they have, and how to best use them.

Chapter 3: Patience

Patience is the foundation of mental toughness, because only through patience can you have spent the time to develop the raw faculties that toughen the mind. You cannot be mentally tough without having done the hard yards. It simply comes no other way and there is no shortcut. Patience alone will soon toughen even the most juvenile of minds, and the absence of patience is easily observed as dilettantism.

Mental toughness is probably about half patience. This fact is excruciating because it ignores your ability to train harder, fit more in, push your limits, and gather more data, and even further than that, it is where you will undoubtedly fail if you don't have enough.

It can even be said that mental toughness at its core is *about* patience more than anything else, because every other factor goes nowhere without it. You can handle all the stress, complexity, competitiveness, confusion, fear, and doubt any sport can throw at you—but it will be your patience that the toughness of your mind will ultimately balance upon.

It's no secret that patience is hard. Especially for the athlete primed over a long time of training for competition and performance, patience is both the thing that gets you through and the thing you will always need to confront. Unlike other things such as perspective and focus, you cannot defeat patience because no matter how patient you become, there will always be things that test it.

This does not, though, equate patience to futility, indeed the opposite. Developed patience is the capacity to see beyond futility, to see that as frustrating as having to wait maybe, waiting out the passing of time is also where things like maturity, respect, and wisdom come from. Put another way—there are things you cannot achieve in the fast lane, and they are the things we often value the most.

Time

Patience is you and all your potential interfacing with the reality of time. maybe at some greater quantum level time itself functions differently, but in the cold hard world of sport, it has all the malleability of concrete. Some things simply require the passage of time to achieve, so all you can do is use it effectively and accept that there will be times when it is out of your hands.

Effective use of time goes a long way to developing patience, by reducing your time being wasted and letting you greet the times when you must be patient as positive. A time that is perceived more clearly can be better allocated, and at its best, orchestrated into timelines that work in conjunction with the timelines of other things like yearly cycles and seasons.

Rising above amateur levels, it soon becomes apparent that the serious athletic process is a matter of working against the timelines of multiple factors. Competitions come in years and seasons, training blocks come in weeks and months, events happen over days, and the basic timelines of life play out as people age and the world changes.

How the athlete relates to these "wheels within wheels" of overlapping timelines is what generates their time-sense and the role patience plays in it. We all want what we want right now, but of course, things don't work like that, so how an athlete deals with the way time is spent is what defines them down the line by the way they have arranged things.

Good athletes know they can only push so far at any one time, or they risk over-extending and delaying recovery after. This is frustrating, and applies to nearly every aspect of athleticism, from strength training to competition cycles, development blocks, and the off-seasons. Patience here is the final factor in the timelines of all sports because once the small percentiles, time envelopes, and schedules have been exhausted, it is what the athlete must face seeing the timeline through. Some things cannot be hurried. The only option is to wait and plan things around these phases to make the most of the time.

Understanding the way time passes within your sport becomes central to the process when the athlete wants to make real changes. Some sports change slowly, with even small changes taking years to enter into practice and years after that before the effects are felt. In these cases, the athlete needs to project the way they intersect with this timeline, i.e., where they are at the start and will be throughout the process. This is big-picture stuff, where the athlete is performing to the greater standards of the sport, possibly dedicating a career to see them through all the stages they must pass. Patience and mental toughness will be critical to this athlete, for the understanding of the time taken and every moment along the way.

Stoicism

You don't need to actually subscribe to being a Stoic to have the patience of someone who does. Stoicism is the capacity to endure the passage of time and the trials that go with it. It is the understanding that all things will pass regardless of how frustrating they may be, and that to grind against time is to grind against the mind itself. In a trite way, this can be seen as going with the flow—and that sometimes the flow isn't going fast enough.

Stoicism has much to offer the athlete because it gives perspective and integrity to the attribute of patience. A stoic mind in itself is a large part of mental toughness because its very essence is being able to endure, control your reactions, accept time as an ever-present element, and give context to your thoughts and communication that has perspective and precedence.

Stoicism brings to mental toughness those things that are often overlooked by the athlete in the process of toughening their mind—all those background attributes that don't have the immediacy and profundity of more overt traits like positivity, focus, and tenacity.

Developing stoicism is the process of applying reason and awareness of yourself within the world, including how time affects all things. To be stoic means to realize that all things have a time element they must abide by, that items cannot be rushed, and that forcing the way things happen will change the outcome. Stoicism is what lets the athlete allow things to simply play out, knowing that their reactions will only alter what may otherwise be a result they want.

Unlike a common misconception about stoicism, it is not to be uncaring or unmoved, instead, it is to be aware enough of what is happening to react with reserve. To the athlete, this means knowing how their sport and preparation intersect, and how some things must be allowed to grow to a certain state of readiness before they can best act. Things like the accumulation of understanding and perspective, the development of endurance, the turnover of teams, the maturity of competitors, and the conditions in which competition takes place, can only arrive at a state to be acted on with an understanding and patience that cannot be pushed.

At its core, stoicism is patience played out in the dynamic and multi-leveled timelines of athletic performance, where the big cycles of competition must be matched to the micro-cycles of preparation, and the whole bandwidth is allowed to speak with a mentally tough enough to wait. This can involve being in the middle of huge processes that are changing fast, but knowing that until critical elements are ready, the best action is to wait. This of course can be extremely difficult, especially when processes have taken years to come together, but the athlete who has developed their mental toughness will have the perspective that rewards their patience.

Chapter 4: Control

Control is what you build mental toughness with, and the result of your efforts is that control you then get to express. Control is both an attribute and an outcome of mental toughness in a loop whereby exercising control in yourself expands your capacity to take control of your circumstances.

Controlling your reactions and responses means controlling their outcomes, and while you can't control all outcomes, you can control your place in them. This is integral to athleticism, which at a deep level is the essence of controlling abilities to have the highest outcomes possible. The athlete that understands and controls themselves to the highest degree can take their performance to levels the athlete who lacks control cannot.

Mental toughness is built on the concept of control. Controlling how your mind makes decisions, controlling how your body focuses its abilities, controlling how you prepare and plan, and controlling the environment—including the people—we perform in, is the fundamental way an athlete shapes their results. Mental toughness is needed here because this level of control across so many aspects, requires focus, perception, and energy to make it competitive. All athletes are doing this, but it is those who exercise control to a higher level that will prevail, which means committing more effort and time than those you compete against

Control in the context of mental toughness does not imply rigidity or an authoritarian attitude to your mindset. If anything, it is the opposite. Real control is the ability to actively influence the greater faculties of the mind, so they do what you require of them. This is a very different thing from having to hammer away for control of a mind that is unruly and ill-contained because this means to control at a deeper level rather than trying to direct things.

Breathing Control

Mental, physical, and reflexive control must include breathing because breathing is how you control your heart rate, and as your heart rate rises, you lose control. Breathing is the bridge between your physical self and your mental self and can be adjusted in all sorts of ways using techniques that stimulate, relax, stabilize, and anchor the body or mind in the way you want to.

At one level, breathing is an integral part of meditation or yoga, where it is used to still the mind and bring it to a state apart from the physical body, but breathing is also a fundamental method used in other sports with a lot of cross over that can be useful for all athletes. Lifters use breathing to create internal pressure to help tension and avoid injury, shooters use breathing to even their heart rate so they can act between beats, swimmers use breathing to affect buoyancy and resistance, and runners use breathing to maintain cardiovascular output.

In fact, most sports will have a breathing element that will be used to enhance their most critical elements and are worth seeking out and developing as these are ways to control different aspects of the mind.

Mental toughness intersects with breath control because these techniques go right to the heart of the mind's ability to be taken into places that are at the extremes of performance. Beyond where bulk ability and conditioning can take an athlete, it is the highly focused control mechanisms like breathing that emerge as imperative skills right at the performing edge.

Breathing control, in some respects, defines mental toughness because it is what anchors mental and physical activity to the situation, and as situations evolve, breathing is like gears that help the athlete's responses shift. The practiced athlete intentionally adjusts their breathing going into a competition, to dispel stress and to ready the body and mind for the sorts of actions required. This may mean keeping the heart rate low to have the body relaxed and the mind open and observant, raising the heart rate to intensify focus and stimulate a fast response, or using certain breathing patterns to engage muscular tension for things like power output or pull strength.

It is this ability to control the mind-body loop that gives the high-performing athlete their confidence as situations escalate, giving them a controllable constant for when all else is volatile. What is often taken as brute resilience is in fact a much finer ability to control the breath and is a perfectly trainable mechanism.

Athletes train breath control by familiarizing themselves with patterns so they become embedded and can be recalled when a situation's dynamics start to rise. This takes time and intentional repetition, and it is common to see athletes forget or disregard their breathing as they become distracted by events. It takes effort and commitment to learn to trust breathing, and good practice means intentionally raising scenarios where the breathing mechanism is used to work out triggers that initiate controlled breathing at the point where the athlete needs it.

This sort of training is often seen in martial arts and rock climbing but can be found anywhere the execution of performance is highly dynamic, such as pitching and track and field. Mental toughness becomes quickly part of this process as the patience and detachment needed to keep returning to the point of stress builds a mind that is structured and confident in itself.

Boundaries

Half the control is not letting your energy and integrity be diverted away by others because you can't control what is beyond your reach. Mental toughness is rooted in knowing and understanding what you can control and what you can't, and responding appropriately and in proportion.

Discerning what is within your control requires boundaries, and those set clearly and intentionally create a secure position in the world. This means knowing what your boundaries are and knowing what happens as you approach or confront them, so boundaries based on quality information, experience, and training create a more stable character than boundaries that are not.

Athletes with vague or badly informed boundaries often do not make it into the higher echelons of competition because they do not have the discipline or security to compete with all the diversity and idiosyncrasies of the international scene. By its nature, to take your sport outside of the local customs and values is to put it up against norms and social factors that will be confronting.

The inverse of this is also true; athletes who can happily face the diversity of the world arena will have fewer impediments to getting there and less stress if they do. By having boundaries that are broader and more inclusive, the process of moving through higher levels of performance consumes less of their energy and mental state. These athletes are often renowned for their apparent toughness and resilience, for being able to live with the rigors of international performance, often for years. Of course, there are many factors that contribute to that, with a major one being that they are clear and comfortable with who they are in fields that are extremely diverse and complex.

Boundaries often cited as important to performance are knowing your acceptable levels for personal interaction, responsibility, intellect, and competitiveness, which means knowing what you are willing to do to prevail. The athlete with high levels of integrity will have boundaries that keep them in the game fairly, inclusively, and with respect, whilst the athlete with weak boundaries will be easily influenced by factors leading to cheating, personal problems, team problems, and ignorance.

You develop your boundaries by discerning how you want to interact with the world and having the personal courage and control to find where your comfort zone ends. The better athlete willingly chooses to push their boundaries beyond their comfort, confront new ideas, enlarge their comfort zone, and reduce the number of things that trigger stress, especially when it is automatic.

Reactions

Reactions define your mindset, and the mind that is in control of as many of its responses as possible is less subject to unwanted actions brought on by stress. Controlling your reactions means being able to choose how to react even when events are happening fast and with a high level of consequence, and the athlete that can do this is less manipulable by external forces, so they exert more of their own control over what they are doing.

For poorly trained athletes, their reactions are usually reflexive and without context, and the very act of conditioning and training is to increase control. As an aspect of mental toughness, controlling reactions is central to the mindset because our reactions are often our weaknesses and we base our mindset on automatic responses that may be outmoded, unrealistic, or even incorrect.

Reactions are controlled by analyzing your own behavior to discern where your control ends, and automatic responses begin. This is done by carefully going through your mental sequences, and slowly going through your physical conditioning, to uncover what you are doing intentionally and what you are not. Uncontrolled reactions are found to be dictating our responses at all levels, often being the product of learning during our formative experiences, which means they may not be useful now. Some reactions will even have been forced upon us, by seemingly arbitrary forces that were present when we first learned or were trained.

Now at one level reactions are important, so long as they are actions the athlete has chosen and developed for the purpose. Reactions that are simply unanalyzed and from unknown origins are vulnerabilities that make an athlete's character both uncontrolled and corruptible. In the face of competition, uncontrolled reactions can be predicted by opponents and exploited, and endurance sports can lead to mindsets that cause the athlete to give up or miss opportunities.

Reactions can be difficult to change because the level of self-evaluation can be invasive as some reactions will form part of our idea of self. It is common to see athletes push back when their reactions are questioned, often seeing this as an insult rather than just a critique of their actions.

Retraining reactions is a good way to improve performance because it goes into the fundamental actions of an athlete that can include subtle problems that affect overall performance. Often, issues that seem impossible to rectify at the overt level are caused somewhere deeper and overlooked, where something as simple as the foot choice an athlete uses unthinkingly, or the way they react to fatigue, thirst, or pressure, sets the rest of their behavior on a course that is hard to control.

Retraining reactions can have pronounced effects because this means taking control at a level that was previously automatic. Sports like tennis, martial arts, motor racing, and gymnastics particularly–sports that have very rapid reaction times–are dedicated to training and conditioning reactions, and these methods can have a lot of overlap with any other sport too.

Chapter 5: Positivity

Positivity is what makes mental toughness inspiring, and without it, mental toughness is merely enduring. The toughest minds out there are not tough because they can suffer through the ordeals they go through—they are mentally tough because they relish it. Your ability to just endure will get you through the season, past selection, or to the finish line, but it is the positivity that makes you sing while you do it and then go the extra mile.

Forget the cliche of the grizzled, cynical, and melancholic "hard man" because that is not necessarily toughness at all, more often being just resignation. The authentically tough mind is the one that sees the good in the situation, strives for progress, not simply closure, and broadcasts positivity that others pick up on.

Positive athletes are not necessarily bubbling over with optimism and jocularity but will have an underlying attitude that recognizes the positivity that is presented and seeks to find it in all scenarios. In the context of mental toughness, this is one of the factors that allow an athlete to stay in the field longer, find solutions where others give up, and give reason to processes that may otherwise be ambiguous.

Mental toughness without positivity becomes cynical and sarcastic, which is self-limiting. Yes, an athlete can carry off a dour or dark persona, but that need not prevent a positive approach to what they do, and can in fact enhance it by giving them a distance from a lot of the "junk positivity" around. In these times, the difference between hype, or the *impression* of positivity, and a genuinely positive attitude can be hard to discern, requiring mental devices such as a dark or intense attitude that rock stars have long used to make clear.

Media

It's OK to feel good, though a huge media sector concerned with portraying mental toughness tends to leave that out. Instead, mental toughness is shown as some sort of intense smugness with a thousand-yard stare, which leaves out the reality of being much more balanced and simply fun.

You won't see 'fun' mentioned much in most of

the information around mental toughness, which is usually concerned with selling products or programs to people wanting to buy an attitude rather than cultivate one. This is a shame because, at the performance edge, where mental toughness matters most, fun is usually a major element and the reason for being there.

The reality is that what most media aims to provide is *satisfaction*, and that is something that need not have a positive effect. Be wary of media that trades on cynicism, popularism, and conspiracy when the sense of satisfaction comes not from attaining something yourself, but instead from detracting from others. Without demonstrating yourself to be better, scathing insults and contrived outrage are nothing more than mimicry and the generation of noise without a signal that does not transmit any positive information. This makes you no more than a re-layer of opinions.

Be careful what you expose yourself to. Some forms of media have more positive content than others, and it is not always apparent superficially which is which. Always keep in perspective that all media is manipulated and that the hype and enthusiasm you see have been contrived to motivate you. There is nothing inherently problematic with this, so long as you keep all media in perspective with what you use it for, and don't draw expectations or conclusions that may not be intended. A good example here is music videos, where minus the music, the visuals change context, and the message is misinterpreted.

Positive People

You become what you hang around, so hanging around positive people is the obvious thing to do. The athlete who is training hard and may have a lot of their life dedicated to the purpose will find conflict with people who do not see this in a positive light. This doesn't mean everyone around you needs to feed directly into what you are doing, but it does mean deciding how much time you spend and the influence you receive from people who don't accept the positivity in your commitments.

Positive people need not have anything at all to do with the sport you do and can provide good interaction that is an alternative to the often narrow world of performance. Having good acquaintances that help you maintain a life that is fun and valuable away from your sport is a big part of making athletic performance sustainable over time.

Hanging around positive people and forming groups with a positive spin on them is part of the greater mindset that lets you decompress effectively so you can reenter performance rested. Because being mentally engaged all the time at a high level runs the risk of burnout, positive social interaction lets you balance things out. This means having social circles that are positive in the moment, but that respect the way serious athletic performance affects your life. Positive friends accept that there will be times when you are fatigued, commit to specific timelines and diets, are there when you are injured, and see you as more than just an athlete.

Of course, group positivity only works when you extend the same to others, and sharing the ins and outs of what everyone is doing provides a healthy social level that gives you more to live than just training and competing. Being positive towards others' goals and processes finds new horizons and broadens what you engage in within the world, which brings valuable insights that fortify the toughened mind.

The finest athletes elevate others because they know their performance gets attention, and with that attention comes responsibility. When you perform at any level that results in being reported or becoming a source of information, you will inevitably have to explain your actions and ideas, and this is where positivity makes a difference. Watch an interview with an accomplished athlete, and you will note that the higher the level, the more their enthusiasm becomes obvious, and the more they realize the details of what they do build the attitudes of the next generation.

Projection

The athlete who projects positivity gets noticed. Being seen to be positive and making situations positive is a basic way to control what is around you. It draws out the potential that attracts the best in others, which in turn keeps things moving forward rather than stagnating.

Being able to project positivity onto an event or performance means being able to cast things in a light that makes them worth excelling at and, therefore, having a quality of achievement that enhances character. We have all known situations that appeared pointless or trivial until a better mind reframed things to make them something desirable and with value. Bringing this to a scenario is a big part of being a good team leader or coach because it makes people trust you.

Projecting positivity is never about over-selling or embellishing. Instead, it is about seeing details and uncovering values that the undeveloped mind lets slip by. Indeed, the truly developed mind is able to extract the details and see the positivity in even the most mundane or negative events, thereby bringing value to something and making it part of their greater experience. Bringing this to sport and athleticism is a way to train better, enter a competition in a better mindset, maintain that mindset throughout difficult aspects of performance, and frame the entire process even if it results in a loss.

This is a tactic used by athletes facing enormous levels of competition like international-level series or multi-events such as the Olympics. Positive projection is how to stage racers in cycling or adventure racing keep their mindset aloft across days of competing, sometimes in the hardest endurance events in the world.

Chapter 6: Growth

You don't get handed mental toughness, you have to grow it. Unlike many things in the athlete's world, you cannot be given, cannot take, and cannot buy mental toughness. Instead, you must nurture it through its stages of growth and give it the direction and conditions to become the attributes of character that will stand up to the rigors of competition and performance when it counts.

When you see mental toughness play out, what you are observing is not the result of 'life hacks' or luck or good looks or portraying an attitude—what you are seeing is the character that is the result of personal growth that does not happen without intent.

Never, ever, think you have arrived. The illusion that you now have all you need to perform is the death of potential and a huge vulnerability to your competition. Mental toughness is greatly undermined by an inability to see the potential in yourself and in a situation because it limits your ability to anticipate and predict. A mentally tough athlete can look at a situation like a game, event, or performance and quickly evaluate the factors that can expand and open up into opportunities they can engage in, rapidly taking on more information to use.

Growth is organic, and everything that grows does so within a niche to lets its potential play out. Mental toughness means knowing the niches you perform within—the sports you choose and the way you compete—and developing your growth to match them. Like all of life, one niche influences another, so smart athletes take lessons from elsewhere and use them to enhance and adapt how they grow for a performance advantage.

Learn to Learn

For many people, learning is a very formal thing that needs to take place within strict parameters such as a school or course, and outside of this, taking on new information can be hard. Given the weaknesses of many modern education systems, this is understandable, but to develop as an athlete the urge and ability to learn needs to be reignited so they can take on the data a modern athlete has available.

For the child, learning is seamless, with little distinction between just living life and taking on the information. Children have little separation between play, learning, and entertainment, and bringing this mindset to adulthood self "softens the wiring" that allows learning new stuff later in life.

It greatly helps to understand how learning happens, so you can stimulate the process and enhance the different phases. The actual details of learning are highly complex and not fully understood, but the basic overview of how we take on information is enough to apply to any body of knowledge, and particularly easy to apply to athletics and sport.

There are four stages to learning:

1. **Unconscious incompetence** is when you don't know that you don't know and the skill or subject matter is alien or not even on your radar.

2. **Conscious incompetence** is when you know there's a void in your understanding and ability, but you have not addressed it. If the uncovering of a missing ability or understanding excites you, then you are on the path to mental toughness as you expand

your horizons. If not, then you are looking at ignorance.

3. **Conscious competence**, is when you know how to do something or have taken on new information and can skillfully execute it with careful preparation and all the right elements. This is to have learned and is a big part of mental toughness because it is the fruit of your effort and shows you have what it takes to develop the capacity to prevail.

4. **Unconscious competence** is what can sometimes appear as talent when really it is the mastery of skills or knowledge, so you embody them. This is the mental toughness you don't even think of as mental toughness, and all the abilities you have that simply make you who you are.

These stages are simple to see at play when learning anything new, and recognizing them greatly enhances the process. When you understand that your brain and body are going through well-defined stages, how you approach what you are learning can be worked with in certain ways.

When you are in the initial phase of not knowing what you need to know about a subject or skill, the objective is to gather as much information as possible, so you have an overview of what is involved. Many people mistake this as actually learning when all it really is, is a collection of data, and as yet nothing has been refined by experience and repetition to even evaluate what will work or not. Knowing what this stage is about–that it is not yet really learning–lets you dismiss any preconceived notions and simply focus on the breadth of the data you collect. At this stage, the more, the better, without prejudice, so you gain more from the next phase.

Knowing you don't know is the state most people walk around in, and in the process of learning is where things can feel the most difficult. This is often associated with sitting bewildered in classrooms or being overwhelmed with complexity, or in the case of athletes, feeling they can never take on what's needed to go to a high level. Without realizing there is much more to the learning curve than this, it is easy to form that mindset, by mistaking the stage of realizing you don't know for the latter phase of realizing you do. Without fully accepting and recognizing what you don't know, and learning afterward, runs the risk of simply being memorization and rote rather than actual understanding.

Being consciously competent, or knowing that you now know, is something most people reserve for only a handful of things in life. Indeed, it can be rare to take on any new avenues of knowledge once in adulthood, which is a shame, and counter to mental toughness. Mental toughness, almost by definition, means being able to take on the rigor of learning to at least this level and developing the ability to exceed the demands of performance.

When you no longer need to focus in order to do things well—when to the observer it will appear as 'effortless' or 'natural'—you will have learned something to the degree that it is now part of your behavior. Of course, this is the goal, and to the athlete, it is where the highest level of performance happens. Because you have learned and assimilated detailed elements of your sport, you can stack newer information you are still processing on top. Your body of ability is broad, so this can be taken on new techniques and ideas that give you a performance edge. Combined, all this is a large part of mental toughness because you simply have a larger base of ability to use, and so situations that confuse or overwhelm the less developed mind to the toughened mind are within its experience.

Any piece of information can be viewed this way, and you have already been doing this your entire life. What makes it integral here is being aware of the process, choosing the stuff you want to know, and cultivating it through the stages of learning intentionally. This is not limited to tangible athletic skills and works the same for abstract or intellectual information. Just as this is how you learn to use a racquet, bike, your legs, or ice tools, this is also how you learn strategy, troubleshooting, timing, and recovery.

Process Before Result

You don't see growth in the mirror. What you see are freeze-frames of growth in the form of subtle results, meaning the 99.9% that is going on when you are not observing yourself is the great process of development you are only partially aware of.

So get aware.

Mental toughness is massively concerned with where you are within any given process, and knowing where you are on the curve determines what specifically you achieve. The mind that is toughened is honest about where they are at, so they can judge performance accordingly to make the most of their ability.

The mentally tough athlete embraces, takes on, and judges themselves and others by the process of learning more so than by the result. What you are doing now, what your teammates and the competition are doing now, is what gives you the ability to predict what your performance will be like on the day. It doesn't matter if today you can run, hit, lift, or push to a certain standard if you don't understand how you got there and where things will go between now and the zero hours of performance.

To the good athlete, any result is nothing more than the outcome of their preparation, with the final performance often being no more than seeing the total process through. especially for endurance events where the build-up can be years, the peak effort actually comes *before*, the final one. It is simply a conclusion where all elements come together.

If you don't love the process, you will find progress haphazard at best and impossible at worst, so it makes sense to build your goals around what you can prepare for. Any result you pursue will have minimum standards and basic skills you need to acquire and master, so you need to have those in perspective to even be a contender and consider any result.

It is common to see a major weakness in an athlete's mindset is their disdain or dismissal of parts of the process they need. Compared to the great athlete who either happily or by discipline or work ethic embraces all the necessary elements, the athlete who doesn't is expecting a result they won't see. Meanwhile, the result they can expect is to be spat out down the line where the energy and time invested stops matching up to the outcome, with athletes having the cause even alluding to them. By not seeing the process clearly, understanding how it relates to the result, and getting on board, performance can be substandard and by then difficult to fix.

Beyond this level of the process is the greater "big picture process," which we have already touched on, and how you engage the total process of your sport and your life. This means being an athlete means fitting in and what you want the greater outcome of all this to be. Do you look beyond your performance years and have the mental toughness to live where all this is behind you? Where can the process go and who will you become?

Chapter 7: Emotional Stability

No emotional stability, no mental toughness. It's that simple. Nothing—*nothing*—hemorrhages away the faculties of the mind like emotions that have no reference, are uncontained, and are allowed to infect other attributes. A stable emotional state is what makes mental toughness reliable and realistic because it keeps the mind from the biochemical whirlpools of turmoil that emotions trick you into.

This doesn't mean the athlete has no emotions, and it certainly doesn't mean they have just buried them under the guise of attitudes and false responses that appear stable and contained. What it means is that the mentally tough athlete knows where their emotions rise from, what effect they have on their character, and how to express them healthily and effectively, so they work for them rather than against them.

Some of the most profound performances have been the result of powerful emotions, harnessed and directed to provide stability rather than erode it. Grief, outrage, despair, joy, and lust have all been channeled as fuel for efforts that, without that extra source of energy, might have been average or meaningless.

Neoteny

The nature of athleticism is to prolong and enhance the state of neoteny—the juvenile state where the body and mind are most trainable, repairable, and reflexes are quickest. This is what lets athletes combine maturity with the benefits of youth, but can also affect their emotional stability with confusing results.

Most athletes get serious in their mid-teens when their bodies are approaching peak ability, and the awareness of performance is rising. The standards abided by here and the general attitude to sport is what will define athleticism for the rest of their lives, but not always are emotions factored in.

It is normal to see sportspeople channel their emotions into their efforts as a way to divert from or ignore emotions they don't like or that don't fit their ideas. This is usually sustainable through till about the early twenties, when it becomes awkward as the pressures and realities of adulthood start to creep through the cracks.

The key here is to know the role emotions play, both biologically and athletically, so you can make them healthy. As alluring as athletic performance may be, it may not be worth a life of painful or discordant emotions that are the result of ignoring them, so the young athlete is encouraged to understand their emotions.

Emotions, of course, are deeply personal, and understanding and expressing them needs the right environment, and the arena of sport has not always been ideal for that. Some sports that take place far from the watchful eye may be better, where groups are the result of a common desire to confront themselves away from a judgmental society. Otherwise, sports can act like pressure cookers, only amplifying and distorting emotional feedback in surges of displaced youthfulness that can be confronting and bizarre.

It is smart to discern what the causes of emotions are, so they can be held distinct from the intellect and rational mind. While being integral, emotions are based on fleeting events, which are good for energizing the mind but not for making important and rational decisions. The goal here is to retain the benefits of emotional energy as a way to keep the mind engaged but to get beyond the juvenile perspective that emotions dictate reality. The power of emotions makes it easy to adhere to this illusion, but by keeping the rational parts of the mind engaged and developed, they give emotions the perspective and gravity they deserve.

Emotional maturity comes when you are responsible for your feelings, and that includes the way they are infused with your sports ambitions. Mental toughness greatly pivots on this, because a mind distorted and exhausted by emotional strain will be unlikely to withstand the duress of higher levels of performance, the confusion resulting only compounding the load.

Getting off the Ride

Emotions are chemical processes that flood your body with compounds to cope with the stresses of powerful situations. The compounds bridge the mind that is inundated with stimulation and messages, and the body that is trying to act. It is not hard to disrupt or manipulate these processes, either to initiate emotions or diffuse them using mental techniques that affect part or all of the process along its continuum.

What can be hard, though, is choosing to control emotions, because the biochemical processes have all sorts of triggers that make them feel important and integral to life. Now to be sure, *some* degree of emotion is fundamental to both living in society and the experience of the sports you have chosen—where would baseball be without the camaraderie, cycling without the surges of the peloton, and climbing without the fear and accomplishment—but emotions themselves are not the experience, they are the product of it.

When emotions become the reason for experience, either consciously or unconsciously, you have entered into a theme park of rides competing for your attention with little control. When the reason for doing something is to have an emotional result, your mindset will be open to any influence that provides it.

This behavior and thinking are just as corrupting either way, either finding satisfaction in the swirl of emotions that come with negativity or being addicted by the lust to win because both allow fleeting sensations and drama to override accomplishment. Over time, like all chemical addictions, tolerance will build, satisfaction will wane, and the drive for the emotional kick will become distorted. This is often seen in athletes who replace the grandeur of winning with grief at the loss, or who take on self-destructive behavior once the hype of the limelight moves on, where the buzz needs to be there in whatever form it comes in.

Mental toughness is impossible with this sort of emotional instability because emotion is out of proportion with other mental attributes like reason and intellect. This means what is essentially a process for expression is diverting energy and attention from processes for the uptake and execution of information. Where mental toughness is built on developing high levels of focus, patience, and control, emotional turbulence undermines all that with unhealthy levels of stress and reaction.

Healthy Emotions

Mental toughness is not to be impervious to emotions, it is to have them in context and proportion, so they express your mental state. The loose and flappable mind is just as dysfunctional as the unfeeling and unexpressive one, as both are undeveloped and without control.

Healthy emotions are not reactions, they are expressions. In this form, they are not uncontrollable responses to situations you are overwhelmed by; instead, they are reasonable expressions of an internal state. Used to express rather than define an athlete's mental state, emotions find their place in the spectrum of faculties and are easier to control because they do not take precedence over those that keep perspectives like patience and detachment.

In this context, healthy emotions become powerful ways to shed tension and stress caused by the strong internal responses that athletic performance brings. Both negative and positive responses can overwhelm the mind with stimulation and information throughout the course of competition and performance, and well-controlled emotions are a way to contain and express that as a release. Healthy emotions are expressed in the context of when they arise, with a clear connection to what causes them, so they do not become distorted and misunderstood. This avoids the common experience of "bottling up" those emotions, where context and timeliness are avoided, so expression becomes about other things that are not always clear.

Emotions expressed in time with events are part of the event, thus giving the context needed to allow healthy release. The ecstasy of winning, the frustration of failing, the anguish of loss, and the wanderlust of reaching new heights, when expressed openly and at the right time, allow the tension of the moment to release as the moment passes. Rather than dragging the stress of the event over to the time when focus and reason are needed, and the stimuli of the event have passed, properly expressed emotions remain part of the timeline in accordance with physical condition and location.

Being psycho-physical, emotions are very much influenced by your physical state, something often overlooked when emotions are high. States of fatigue, low blood sugar, innervation, sleep deprivation, and sudden opportunities to relax can all bring on emotional surges as the chemical relationship between the brain and body changes. Very often, acute emotional experiences are dictated more by these factors than any other, but if not recognized, they become reacted to as something else.

It is vital to the athletic mindset to know when emotions are being exaggerated by purely physical factors, so that they can be both understood and controlled. Awareness of diet and calorie intake, hormonal balance, stress levels, and fatigue status means you can anticipate your emotions so they won't have a confusing impact. This really matters in groups, where the emotional failings of one member can disrupt everyone else, especially in things like endurance events or competitions where the team is in close contact for a long time. When the breakdown of team dynamics is catastrophic, emotions become as big a feature as ability and group role, and healthy expression matters as much as other attributes of personal performance.

Relationships

Nowhere else are emotions felt more than in relationships, with interpersonal interactions potentially viewed as "emotion generators." Alone, emotions can be epic enough, and with the addition of other people, things can become dynamic and dramatic.

We all know this, and some people are better at stabilizing their emotions with other people than others, seemingly unflinching and unfazed by how two humans interplay. When expressed well, emotions become the bond of a group or partnership, making them a powerful tool for forming good teams to compete with.

Group emotions have long been known as a good way to focus and strengthen a team, cultivating group expression with things like team rituals and shared experiences. The team that wins together stays together, bonding over more than sports performance, but the shared emotion of prevailing can last longer than the event.

This same paradigm stands for partnerships—in sport and in life—and the athlete with healthy emotional expression in one will have it in the other, and likewise the opposite. Emotional turmoil dragged from one world to the other, such as family or work over to athletic performance, can have volatile results.

But we do not live in perfect worlds, things happen, and at some point, the chance of emotional upheaval is pretty much guaranteed. Relationships have their troubles, people change, work will have its issues, circumstances take twists and turns, and in these times it is imperative the athlete knows how to channel strong emotions into performance or they risk being swamped by them.

This is where all this becomes important, because the athlete with the right degree of mental toughness will be able to channel these strong emotions into their training and performance and turn them into something productive, probably like no other avenue will allow. Athletes fueled by grief, anger, and contempt can divert these feelings from being self-destructive or even problems for others, and turn them into performances where remarkable things happen.

This takes real fortitude, perspective, tenacity, and detachment and is the sign of a mind truly strengthened, but is something bigger than merely a sporting accomplishment. The ability to do this in the context of relationships can turn all the volatility of interpersonal interactions, even among strong characters, into inspiring and accomplishing partnerships. Examples of this are maybe not common, but profound when they emerge, of people who have high emotional responses but, in the right relationship, become super-capable. This is often seen in pro teams with emotionally charged coaches who bring out the athlete's best, endurance teams who can focus on extroverted characters to overcome extreme fatigue and pressure, and racing teams where strong emotions become a team identity that is formidable to the opposition with their esprit de corps.

Chapter 8: Self-Validation

Self-validation's role in mental toughness is defining who you are, and what you are doing so you can find your place in a scenario. This is the aspect of your mind that asserts that what you are doing is worthwhile, and that carves out your position in the world of competition.

Mental toughness demands a high level of self-awareness and validating the value of your efforts and the way they form your character is part of this. To be resilient through the ordeals of competition, long training, and development of your skills, and the possible years it may take to be at your performing best, it is vital to be clear that what you are doing is worth all the effort and that the athlete you are is clearly defined.

Of course, there will be periods of dissatisfaction and questioning, and the stronger the concept you have of yourself and what you are doing, the less vulnerable you are to the naysayers and the well-meaning who may not simply understand your conviction. Robust self-validation is what lets you separate your actions from being selfish, and what frames your commitments as having more worth than simple self-satisfaction.

Visualization

Visualization techniques are what put you firmly in the game, knowing what you are doing and how you are doing it. Far from the new age version of internally visualizing yourself relaxing or absorbing energy, athletic visualization is the process of running and rerunning through method and performance, so you neutrally embed details that will playback at the sharp end.

These techniques have been around for decades, even centuries with martial arts, and train the mind with a clear picture of the athlete in the continuum of performance. The self-validation aspect is definitive because this is where all of an athlete's ideas about themselves are both formed and reworked and retrained when they are found to fail in the cold light of performance.

The athlete who effectively uses visualization develops a clearer perception of their ability and identity than the athlete who only trains tangibly in the real world. This clearer picture of the self then allows the athlete to compare how they stack up against others and the environments they perform within, building an identity based on clarity rather than assumption.

We all know the risks that basing our identity on assumptions can bring, leaving too much to vagueness and untested ideas. Visualization allows athletes to cut through this habit and to get to know themselves so that they can develop their abilities closer to the actual demands of their sport.

Visualization to do this takes a form similar to meditation, except instead of focusing on the mind, the objective is to focus on the body and mind combined in action. The process is similar to being somewhere without distraction, so the athlete can go deeply into their actions and observe the tiny details.

Like meditation, this is something that takes practice and time, as well as testing in the real world in international circumstances to find out the efficacy. Sports science has taken this process to a very high level, with a large body of research into techniques and effects. At an elite level, things like float tanks and brain function monitors, analyze neural activity to enhance the process. Of course, most athletes have no access to this, but the actual practice still remains, that of spending time running and rerunning actions through the mind, to wire in pathways that will be used during a performance.

What Other People Think

We like to say we don't worry about what other people think, but in reality, this is both untrue and pointless. What matters really is being concerned with what other valuable people think, and the mentally tough athlete is one that is good at discerning this.

Now, it is true that none of us should worry much about petty or trivial reactions from others, simply because at a level of little consequence, mental energy is better spent elsewhere. It is not worth the distraction to be concerned with the thoughts of others if those thoughts would make no difference if you weren't aware of them. In fact, letting these sorts of things concern you is actually to become concerned about your *own* thoughts, now you have taken them on.

The key here is to have a simple indicator of when someone else's opinion of you is not worth regarding, then have the discipline to dismiss the opinion as quickly as it arises. A good indicator can be to gauge if the energy and effort to confront the opinion are greater than what the opinion implies, and if so, the numbers simply don't balance.

Dismissing the opinion of others when it is not worth the energy to confront need not mean completely dismissing them as people or even their opinions on other things or at other times. This is simply a way to filter your own conduct with the many other people you share a world with, where there is limited energy available to put towards the things you must do, including your athletic pursuits.

At the other end of the spectrum are the people you should heed the thoughts of. These can be people who have a pivotal influence on the things you do, or people whose opinions you trust and respect. This ties into the choices you make for those you spend your time with, and you do not have to overtly like these people and their opinions, but you do need to see them as worth learning from.

Examples here are the classic mentor-student relationship, where someone with proven ability and experience imparts it to those willing to learn with a degree of detachment that allows them to avoid commenting on behavior. This way establishes why the relationship exists, something imperative to shared respect, and that the role of the mentor is the development of the student.

This mentor relationship need not be formal, and can happily exist among friends and teammates, the key being the understanding that the objective here is growth and development of the self. Without this clear identity becomes vague and opinions can be construed as insults rather than critiques.

It will always be true that at times we confront what we hear about ourselves that we don't like, and so choosing who we listen to is important. We do not need to be close friends necessarily, but we do need to know that the opinion is both valid and with the right intentions. These intentions, ideally, are for our own growth, but neutrality is also valuable because it applies even outside the context of the relationship, having no bearing on future repercussions thus making it ultimately valuable in the moment.

Self-validation is a large part of what informs mental toughness; it's how effective we are through the eyes of others. Trusted opinion, either from people we are close to or people with no investiture in our process, gives us insight into ourselves we cannot get any other way. This will not always be easy but it directly confirms our mindset by how we respond, and how we structure our ideas about ourselves when we interact with others.

Chapter 9: Tenacity

Tenacity is like the vanguard of mental toughness, the aspect of the character that projects what your mindset is applied to. This attribute is often likened to *will*, but it is so much more than that, being the intersection of the mind's intent and the body's actions.

Alone, tenacity appears as toughness because it is overt and easily noticed by others, but without all the other elements to fortify it, it is just a paper tiger. Real tenacity is the part of being mentally tough that keeps you in the game, not just to perform but to prevail. It is the part of your character that accepts that burning lean tissue will be needed, and the part of you that will go as far as is needed and a bit more just to do it right.

Tenacity does not mean being gung-ho or cavalier, though. Where those traits are loose on reason and subject to emotional instability, tenacity is focused, controlled, and informed. Tenacity forms an integral part of mental toughness because this, as it is how the mind chooses to act on its objectives, then sticks to the plan with confidence.

Developing tenacity can be an exciting part of athletic and personal development because it involves doing all the things that push an athlete to succeed. Only by repeatedly pushing at the edge of performance, then pulling back to assess and adjust, can we see where tenacity needs to be applied and how we can work on it.

At a very superficial level, this seems to be what *all* athletic training is about, but the smart athlete realizes that as valuable as tenacity is, it is not enough by itself. Tenacity needs to be applied effectively, to the things where it makes a real difference, because the energy and focus it requires are too intensive to spread everywhere. It is a common folly to see athletes being tenacious and intense about every aspect of their sport they can find, only falling into mediocrity because they were not distributing their energy, resources, attention, and control discerningly. If anything, athletes like this can simply undermine themselves by lacking depth and periods of recovery.

What this means is that a good athlete learns what tenacity is made up of, and what, from the spectrum of things, they should apply it to. Observing high-level athletes, it is apparent that they reserve their full attention and effort for some things, but elsewhere they take things easy, or even lackadaisical, so as not to burn out.

Will, Resolve, Resilience, and Enduring

Mental toughness gets its teeth from tenacity, which alone is a great attribute to have, and in concert with all these others can be hero-like. That said, tenacity can be poorly defined or substituted with other attributes, and it pays to have them clear in your mind so you can apply each in its best form.

> Will is what you think, tenacity is what you do.

> Resolve is seeing the event through, tenacity is making it on your terms.

> Resilience is holding on, tenacity is the energy you apply.

> Enduring is not giving up, tenacity is not giving up on doing better.

Will is an important attribute to have because it focuses on your choices. This is where what you decide to do—or not to do—goes from being just a notion to being something you get behind. Willfulness is often cited as a fundamental aspect of figuring out your position in the world, with entire philosophies being built around it as a way to get to the core of your experience.

Will becomes tenacity when it becomes an athlete's focus. Even in the face of failure, when despite setbacks and hardships that would otherwise see a change in direction, they choose to persevere. Unlike sheer stubbornness, which is having a disregard for reason and perspective, tenacity is when new courses of action are applied but still to the same objective.

Will directs all this energy, but it is tenacity that actually turns the wheels where the energy is spent. Tenacity is like the vehicle of will, where the calories are burned, and the athlete goes into overdrive. This is where the athlete, for all their motivation, focus, and intent, keeps the momentum alive to get the result already chosen.

Resolve is where the athlete denies any other option other than to carry their efforts through to the end of the plan, and tenacity is to do so not because it's expected but because the athlete has their own reasons. Tenacity here is about controlling performance right the way through, despite it being possible to simply fulfill the standards already set out. This is the athlete doing things on their own terms, and those terms being to a better standard and are where the finest performances exceed the norms.

Resolve is never just a shallow commitment to expectations, it is a full commitment to personal knowledge that this is a time for the athlete to give their best. Tenacity is the additional factor where the athlete plays by standards they choose themselves, that are higher, broader, or even previously unacknowledged.

This level of performance is where the leading edge of sport happens. This is the player who pushes to double the previous winning margin and redefines what a high score means, or the ultra-endurance athlete who pushes without sleep to smash hours off the record. These are the nuts and bolts of athletic evolution, where athletes remaster the way performance can go and change the way things are done.

Resilience is a core attribute to bring to any pursuit, but without tenacity, it can be no more than simply clinging on through pressure. Resilience alone is not enough to out-compete others, it needs the energy and control of tenaciousness to go from being passive to engaging.

Weathering the stresses and difficulties of athletic competition is fundamental at all levels of sport, and the greater capacity for it, the further the athlete can go into the higher echelons where it defines the game. Resilience is needed for the athlete to keep their head through times of pressure when other, easier options may appeal, and the capable athlete will keep on track with their goals. The difference tenacity makes is shifting the process, so the athlete no longer clings to the process, but changes the process by being stronger, more focused, more aware, and more engaged.

The athlete doing this is not just surviving the process but controlling it, using their energy and expertise to intentionally make themselves better at the game. Where the lesser athlete is just sticking with the process as it is, the mentally tough athlete is adapting themselves to find advantages in the difficulties.

Resilience like this has a place in all forms of competition and at every level and is often the factor that sees some athletes progress further than others. Where standard performers are happy to just move through the stresses of training and competition, elite athletes see these stresses as their chance to excel. Accumulative over years, this tenacious attitude to seek advantages where others seek only to persevere is a key component of high-end sports performance. This is the boat crew who trains in harder weather, the swimmer who swims more months of the year, the climber who pushes himself to more remote areas, and the gymnast who adds extra conditioning to.

Enduringness, as opposed to *endurance* which has its own meaning in sport, means staying in the game longer, and tenacity is when you stay longer as a means of prevailing. Where the good athlete has the capacity to stick things out for hours or days, the athlete with superior mental toughness has the capacity to stick it out longer as a standard.

In ordinary life, enduring matters as a way to build capacity and volume, and is the attribute that lets you set your limits far down the line. In athleticism, this becomes something more than just getting the time in, and becomes its own factor as a standard by which you out-perform and win.

Obviously, endurance sports make this their precinct, where the athlete who can endure more time at a greater level of intensity wins, but most sports will have an element of endurance even if it is mostly in training. Tenacity here is when the athlete sees that enduring is essentially the basis of all performance and of fitness itself, and so makes it an attribute they use to prevail. By training better for longer, staying in the game for longer, and developing their capacity to train furthermore efficiently, these athletes have higher thresholds that result in better performance.

Enduringness with tenacity as a select strategy brings some of the biggest performance gains of any methodology, not just because of the larger base of capacity, but because few athletes invest in it, thinking there are shortcuts or the effort is wasted. This is understandable in the amateur and rookie fields, where the experience level is low and time in the sport isn't enough to see beyond anomalies, but step things up to higher levels or sports where the field is bigger, and it fast becomes clear that tenaciously choosing enduringness is where the difference between good and great lies.

The great cosmic joke that comes with this is that by the time the differences are being seen, the window to catch up is fast closing, and those who thought they could beat enduringness with 'hacks' and fast-tracking are missing the attributes that count. This is where the national level performer leaves behind the state level and international level beyond that. This is where tenacity applied smartly across an athlete's career pays off with a tenaciousness in competition those who dismissed it cannot know.

Always a Little Further

Tenacity and mental toughness, in the deepest sense, mean being able to take things further than the forces you oppose. This doesn't mean more than what is thrown at you, but *choosing* to go further against whatever it is. Whether it's against competitors, the weather, previous times, or standards set by others, it means not merely exceeding these things by providence but doing so by design.

Going further is not being opportunistic. Instead, it means putting things on your own terms to go as far as you can take them by choice. This real tenacity is what separates the athletes who prevail over the opposition and those athletes who prevail over the competition itself, and is the highest form of athleticism there is.

At this level, mental toughness is the defining factor in an athlete's capability, and tenacity is both what gets them there and what will see them through. This is where the extra hours, the extra intent, the extra information to draw from, and the extra clarity of the self-performing come together, and tenacity pulls them all through the dynamic of the event.

Later, in the cold light of analysis, this will be seen as the will and presence of mind to push up to 'eleven' and "bring it all home," both cliches that are overused, but in this case, aptly describe the point where tenacity overrides all other attributes.

The illusion, though, is that this will happen to any athlete in the same intersection of time and events, that by some kind of magic they will find a higher gear when things really matter most. But hindsight tells another story in the logbooks of those who don't prevail, finding no other level awaits those who lacked tenaciousness in preparation.

"To go further, you must go further," the creed of the ultra-runner states, and even though preparation is based on a huge body of precision, reasoning, patience, stability, and temperance, the only way to make exceeding the standards part of your reality is to do it. Yes, tenaciousness needs to be applied with reason and clarity, but when it is called for, it must be expressed for what it is.

In the imagination, this ideal of tenacity pushing out to prevail is what many athletes base their entire perspective and process on. The idea that the time will come when everything is on the line, all bases are filled, and the fundamental will to win is what will make the difference. The reality is, if that ability is not there, to begin with, no amount of tenacity can draw on it to push through. In this instance, even the toughest mind makes no difference—perhaps other than confronting the failure afterward–because tenacity now is only the sum of the tenacity that has come before.

What this means to the athlete is to look at your process, the competition, and the training, see where tenacity makes a difference, and focus it there. To a ball player, it may mean pushing precision and strategy late into the game. To the runner it may mean optimizing on the hills and the later miles. To the mountaineer it may mean coping with another night on the mountain.

Chapter 10: Acceptance

There will always be things beyond your control, and it is not enough to simply dismiss them. True mental toughness is the capacity to accept what you cannot prevail over and to face up to what your limitations are.

Acceptance is also to not fall into the cliched junk psychology of "do or die" and "no Plan B," because they are unrealistic fantasies contrived by people who have never performed for real. Without accepting that sometimes there will be failures and defeats, you cannot see the parts of your character that need to grow fast and become discernible as ignorance.

Acceptance is not a convenient way out of failure though—to accept you must take responsibility and it is perhaps here that you will find some of the greatest tests of mental toughness. The things you can accept are the measure of you, even more than your wins and best efforts, which are arbitrary, because what you can accept shows the depth and breadth of what your mindset can tolerate.

The further you go into competition and performance, the more there is to accept, and the untrained mind that finds acceptance difficult will be distracted, unfocused, and wasting energy. Often "the pressure of competition" is exactly this—the limits of what an athlete can accept as their reality—ending some careers prematurely not because the athletic ability was met but because the mind could not keep up.

An inability to accept locks the mind into a loop of reaction that is built on hardwired ideas the athlete can't—or won't—control. To continue to pursue performance the smart athlete knows this is an advantage over those who cannot develop mental toughness and addresses this element of their mindset like any other faculty.

The mind that can accept simply goes further because it has further to go. It stops seeing limitations where there are none and makes the athletic challenges more tangible. On the scale of the factors that make up mental toughness, acceptance is one of the easiest to address because it is so general. Developing acceptance across the greater scope of life has huge overlap and cross-reference to athleticism and sportsmanship, and raises the athlete above merely being good at their sport.

Where You Have No Control

There are always things you cannot control, and how you approach them is a measure of you. Perceiving everything beyond your grasp as a threat or not your problem is the first sign of a small mind that is contained, vulnerable, and hard to work with, and the athlete's attitude to accepting these things is basically an indicator of their limitations.

The unaccepting mind is difficult to place in a team, constantly needing special attention to work around and appease. This makes those who cannot develop limited not just in themselves, but it makes it hard to mentor and relate to those who have performed at these higher levels where acceptance is fundamental.

Accepting where your control ends means accepting a world of competition that is varied and diverse, and the mentally tough athlete approaches this with the excitement of acceptance, not disdain. The toughened mind sees the edge of their control as the frontier of its performance, beyond which they must accept, adapt, and grow to enter. Especially in sports truly on the global stage like soccer, athletics, swimming, cycling, and adventure sports, athletes having a mind that can cope with the breadth of humanities diversity and ideas is integral to pursuing at the higher levels

To go to these levels of performance, the athlete's mind needs to be adaptable to letting go of their own cultural niche and its values and state of control, so it can accept the scale of competition and the basics of simply traveling. For the athlete just entering this level of sport, these things may be confronting, with a kind of "culture shock" as they are exposed to the way international level athletes work.

Letting go of your own values to accept something more diverse is an indicator of a mind that has developed and toughened. It does not mean rejecting or dismissing previous values. Instead, it means placing your own values in context with others and seeing value in the differences.

This is a true test of mental toughness, and not all athletes are up to it, as the realities of competing globally are complex and demanding. It takes a mind that can cope with fundamental challenges in logic, language, attitude, patience, and perspective to stay at this level long enough to matter, but the athletes that are up to it are those who will perform their sport at its best.

The athlete who develops their mind to accept, and welcomes the realm beyond their control finds a scope of capabilities that is beyond the self-imposed limits of the mind. This athlete knows how others do things, including perceiving them. They are the product of their own development, and like all people, they are somewhere along the curve of developing their minds.

The very essence of competition is to match up to where control ends, to prevail against others or conditions at the edge of an athlete's abilities. We can control up to the point where our preparation extends, but beyond that, we must accept we have to adapt and grow, letting go of our own values to take on those that are higher.

When You Can Do Better

Accepting that you have limitations and that the best performances happen beyond the edges of them, means accepting that you can always do better. The athlete who is mentally prepared will see this as an exciting invitation, to grow, let go of their former limitations, and enter a new level.

Knowing how and what you can do better means seeing the athletic process only ends where the mind cannot go, and that is the greatest challenge to mental toughness there is. For all the training and discipline, even for the finest athletes in their field, it is accepting what they can do better that puts them at the vanguard.

The spectrum of things that can be done better is usually complex and wide, and accepting it all takes courage and perspective, but the opportunity to become the best athlete possible makes it compelling. All athletes can usually prepare better with more refined training, advancing their mindsets, and better allocation of resources, and the better ones accept this.

It is important to constantly evaluate your process, not just of training and competing but for life around it. The people you interact with, like family, friends, and at work, will all intersect with your athletic capacity, so they need to be included. The things you can do better at these levels reflect on your performance, and accepting and understanding this is what forms the stability athletes need to perform long term.

Accept that other people have their own limitations and perspectives, every bit as valid and valuable as your own. Accept that circumstances are subject to unique factors of which you are only one among many and that finding what you can do best will influence the whole. Most importantly, accept that where you are now is always at the point of change, and doing things better means doing things differently.

Forgiveness

True mental toughness is a mind that accepts diversity and change because that means you are part of more of the world. Inversely, to have only a narrow degree of acceptance makes you at most the champion of some little niche with no title to claim as anything other than a parochial voice.

The athlete that has chosen to pursue performance to a serious level will come to interact with many different people and reasons along the way, and not all of them will be in their favor. The nature of competition and performance is dynamic, and advantages will always be sought, including at times when they hurt others, and where reason doesn't make sense.

The only smart way to deal with this is to forgive.

Forgiveness doesn't mean submission, condonement, or agreement. What it means is to let go of the need to be vindicated. Sometimes the only resolution is to accept that things happened, that the limits of reason and integrity were found, and that beyond that, there was no perspective that worked. Rather than keep trying to make the past fit, put it to rest with the better values you have now.

Forgiveness works because it happens entirely on your terms. Where someone or a situation has conspired against you, forgiveness retakes the initiative by being of better values and perspective than the event that took place. Forgiveness means acceptance, but it may not mean forgetting, and the mentally tough person does not conflate the two. The old idea that forgiveness is an act of submission is wrong, and when done effectively, is a powerful way to reset boundaries and emotions to improve going forward.

Chapter 11: Attitude to Failure

The dirty secret of mental toughness is that it is riddled with failures because it is your ability to get back up again that is toughness defined. Any fool can assume they are tough when they have never found out what happens to themselves when they hit their limits, and as the old saying goes, "only those who have gone too far know how far they can go."

Mental toughness requires failure, so it knows what resilience and humility are, and so the pains of not prevailing can be seen for the illusions they are. So long as failure is the bogeyman that makes you avoid ever truly pushing your limit, you will in fact be failing constantly until you overcome the greatest point of failure there is—to not commit. Mountaineers have the concept of "training to fail" seemingly an oxymoron, where they attempt peaks knowing full well that summiting is unlikely and they will be turning around early. The lesson here is that success is something bigger than a summit, or a finish line, or the highest score or fastest time, and that getting stuck on trivial failures blinds an athlete to bigger possibilities.

All failure needs to be cast in the light of *what is it that has failed*. Without this analysis of the event, failure can become confusing or misdirected, and the process of trying again is ineffective. Indeed, failing once at something is essentially just part of any process, but failing again, in the same way, shows that the failure itself was something overlooked.

Failure that is looked at with reason and perspective clarifies to be seen for the elements it really is, instead of a single monolithic event that may be lacking in understanding. This process of dissecting and looking at failures in different lights, perhaps with the input of others, is what lets athletes keep their failures in context and proportion.

Analyzed intentionally, failure becomes simply circumstances and the progression of events, and the factors that failed can be pinpointed and addressed. This offers deep opportunities for the athlete to look into their behavior, choices, and potential, instead of accepting failure as being simply "things didn't work."

Failing as Learning

To never fail is to infer that nothing was attempted to a degree that makes a difference. While failure is never explicitly intended, it should always be planned for as a healthy part of athletic preparation. This is the way to include failing in the learning process, by accepting its place in the big picture, so when the time comes—and no one avoids it forever—it is not without perspective, and can be resolved quickly.

Consider that 'learning' is the process of making new connections between logic and reason, and that failure sits within this paradigm. Most obviously, failure shows when logic and reason have not been resolved, but when analyzed closely, it will be shown that for *anything* to occur, logic and reason were in place—but were simply not aligned with intentions to the desired result.

Athletic failures come in various forms, such as losing to competition, not finishing events, inadequate preparation, and misapplied efforts that didn't bring results. None of these things fail without reason, and the subsequent failure may be the only opportunity to look into the machinations of performance, that would otherwise be unobserved, being unnoticed from winning.

Indeed, there are many aspects of elite performance that are *only* accessible by failure, aspects out on the edge of human performance that can only be uncovered by taking the specifics of athleticism to extremes. It is well known in athletics, especially in endurance and team events, that failing within acceptable parameters is the only way for these athletes to attain the perspective and control needed through experience.

The old adage of "success comes from experience, and experience comes from failure" is exactly this, because there is no other way to delve into the complexities and lessons of threshold performance—even by winning or prevailing. The very stuff that appears as magic or unique talent, is only understood through the trials of failing, right out at the limits where an athlete's present understanding ends. Put in another cliched form, "to find the edge, you must go over it."

At this point of failure, it is a sign of mental toughness to maintain awareness and perspective as things miss their mark. Rather than collapsing into the drama of failing, the greatest opportunities for learning are present right as they occur. In these headiest and most extreme moments, as success slips from the athlete's grasp and the new reality of failure presents, the athlete who stays on their game, keeps themselves engaged, and prepares for "Plan B" is always preparing to win the next time around.

This is why mental toughness matters, to never give in even as things fail, and to keep the mindset engaged so that even when you fail at performing, you are not failing to learn. This separates the elite performer from the rest and is a common factor in the stories of most great athletes, who never miss the chance to learn even when things didn't go to plan.

Mental Strategies

"Failure is not an option" is one of the dumbest cliches floating around the world of sports. The obvious element of failure is, of course, unrealistic because to compete at all is to risk failure, but more insidiously is this meme's denial of options.

Every sport and athletic pursuit has its own unique strategies that require a form of thinking and focus. Sports with time limits specialize in optimizing how the clock is used, sports depending on physical strength and speed are dedicated to lining everything up for perfect recruitment, team sports have myriad strategies for the countless possibilities of many people on a field, and endurance sports have strategies to cover things like eating and sleep deprivation—and like gamblers, everyone thinks they have the strategy that will win.

Of course, most strategies don't win, and if they all did, there would be no competition, so what makes one strategy better than another?

The best strategies redefine failure, not to dismiss it under some other guise that sounds nicer, but to open up the mechanisms that lead to it so as to analyze where within their strategy, failure fits in. Failure can very well be the result of planning to win, but getting the context wrong and overlooking factors that were assumed to be solid. This is common, and something acknowledged in all forms of risk management, so every strategy an athlete uses should view all factors equally.

Nearly every failure is met with the response of "I thought I had it sorted," meaning there was nothing out of the blue or unforeseen involved, that what went wrong was right before you but didn't register to be addressed. This is the failure of strategy.

There are always options—including failure—and to discount or deny any is to have gaping holes in your strategy. In effect, this intentionally creates a blind spot, which goes against the good practice in every sport there is. Talk to any high-level athlete, adventurer, or soldier, and they will tell you they strategize every possible angle and run the possibilities, including those possibilities around failure.

Chapter 12: Preparation

Mental toughness is nothing more than the sum total of your preparation. It is the quality and volume of your preparation that determines your mindset, and if that quality and volume pertain to mental toughness, then you will have it, and if it doesn't, you won't.

Preparing to be mentally tough is a big part of any serious athlete's process because it is a fundamental element of performance success. All the hours and routines and details and repetition and experimentation that preparation consists of refining the pillars of mental toughness like judgment, discipline, and patience.

In an often overlooked way, preparation is important for dispelling the illusion that elite performance comes from genetics or some innate talent, because whatever those things contribute, without preparation they mean nothing. Preparation is the simple equation that shows that applied effort is what athletic success is made of, and nothing trumps that, and that mental toughness is therefore as available to you as it is to anyone else. Likewise, the inverse is also the case—lack of mental toughness equates to a lack of preparation, with the solution being nothing more special than the application of effort.

Preparation for the Unpreparable

Beyond the limits of what you know is where real athleticism begins. If all performance was simply to fulfill what an athlete already knows they can do, the sport itself would stagnate and go nowhere. Instead, it is through the dedication of serious athletes that the standards of all sports performance are exceeded, pushing into ability, capacity, strategy, and mindset previously uncharted.

Mental toughness is the deciding factor here because to take things to where no athlete has taken them before demands sustained, smart, and creative preparation, potentially for years. To go into this paradigm, first, the athlete needs to discern what the limits are, what makes their limits, and why no one else has yet gone beyond them. Some things simply need time, for subsidiary factors to be pushed beyond and resolved first, while other things will need redefining and reframing.

Shifting an objective to preparable from being previously unpreparable, is no small thing, and might involve a massive refocusing of athletes thinking, training, and ideas. This is tantamount to taking something that is impossible, pulling it apart, and reconfiguring all the elements so they can be prepared for and consolidated. There is no illusion that the risk is high, but for those with the mental strength to choose it every step off the path of the known is a success. As the motto of the elite Special Air Service regiments plainly states, "Who Dares Wins."

Where logic and precedent start to wane, creativity takes over, and the way previously unattainable objectives have been reached has always involved this. To approach a goal with no existing method of preparation means finding new ways to prepare and develop, as indeed the inverse will not work—to repeat what is known not to work will not change the outcome.

Examples here are many, with famous examples coming from sports like climbing, distance running, skiing, and rugby, where entirely new forms of preparation entered the mix and rapidly shifted what was possible. New ways to train the body according to revised principles, new equipment and ways to use it, new strategies to orchestrate it all, and new types of people entering the field, made new gains attainable and gave rise to even new goals.

Creativity without mental toughness is impossible. This is not the trivial dabbling in amateur attempts, instead, here it means the business of looking deep into the athlete's motivations and abilities and reforging them in a new design. The metaphor is closer to sculpture in marble than to casually scribbling on a napkin, and creativity here involves commitment and burning lean tissue.

This sort of preparation takes the athlete off the standard course and onto one that is parallel to what everyone else is doing, which needs a level of mental toughness that doesn't come by chance. Not every sportsperson either wants or is up to the rigors of forging a new path, and it will test relationships, focus, self-validation, and positivity to their full extent.

Preparing for the unpreparable is the course to take for the athlete already well embedded in the process of aiming for high goals because they will already be familiar with the sharp sting of failing, then trying again. This is the athlete who has reframed success and failure for maximum growth, and who is not afraid or repulsed by the ordeals of personal reconfiguration, understanding that the athlete who succeeds at the previously unattainable is made differently.

To hold this ideal is to fully embody the sport, to be in the game itself in order to change it. Along with many, many quiet but brilliant athletes who pushed what their sport meant, this is also the realm of the most famous by which modern sports are known.

At its most foundational level, this mentality and ability to prepare is about seeing where a sport can go. This is the mental toughness to question what currently exists, long before the other attributes of redirection training and performance, and it includes flying in the face of traditions and conventions. Many athletes think they have mental toughness already—endowed by being faster, sweatier, or tolerating more pain—yet only the few who sweat, bleed, and gasp in the attainment of something new, really know what toughness is able to bring.

Preparing. *Really* preparing

If you train like everybody else, you will get results like everybody else.

The secret to elite performance is to train secretively. This doesn't mean working behind closed doors. What it means is to use methods unique to yourself, to eschew standardized programs, and to use techniques and methods to put you in a paradigm the opposition cannot expect.

The basis of all training is tried and tested methods—but performed and applied to extraordinary levels. Ninety percent or more of the training that leads to definitive performance is exactly what everyone else does, simply done better and in more volume. The great hitter still punches out hours in the cage, the great runner still puts down the miles on their legs, and the great tennis players all spent the hours on the court, but what makes them different is the paradigm they do it in.

To prepare for goals beyond the norm means maintaining the goal as the omega point towards which all preparation channels. Unlike standard training, which is led by what the athlete is told they must do according to past performance, elite training sees that as only a base. High-level training shifts the source of information in front as an attractor, using a high degree of insight and research into the goal to inform their training instead of only established information.

Beware of forcing preparation to fit the curve of an objective, something that is a common but underlying reason for failure. This means not falling into the trap of plotting from where you are now, to where you need to be at a given time, with a nice even curve upon which you expect all progress to fit. This is folly because it puts faith in an abstract logic that runs counter to what actually governs performance, which is the aforementioned omega point.

The informed athlete, with a developed level of mental toughness, avoids this trap by reviewing their ability to train and prepare from the past, then projecting it into the future, tweaked with any new information they have. This lets them view what is possible according to logic and reason, and *only then* can objectives be planned for with a margin of certainty.

The hidden logic here is how well their past preparation has been—something that is best judged by failures, not wins. In fact, to never have really failed (as detailed in Chapter 11) suggests that you have not been preparing at your optimum, sabotaging future efforts from a lack of quality data.

This form of preparation implies the long game, something by now any athlete should know is a given to performance. Short-term performance may well allow for stunts that *appear* to be ability, but which are in fact simply anomalies that come with the overlap of circumstances. Athleticism is littered with these cases, of seemingly revolutionary performers who rise to attention with a single performance but disappear as 'one-hit wonders' because they lack true forward vision.

To change the field and perform at a new level, it is necessary to strip all the novelty and stunt-work out of preparation and address the process at its core for its efficacy in making deep changes. We already know that standard athletes do not produce extraordinary outcomes despite occasional anomalies, that are the product of the sport, not exotic new elements.

Avoid the trap of loading your training and preparation with a bunch of weird elements simply because they are exotic. That is to dabble in the unfounded at best and can be an outright scam at worst. Instead, program your preparation based on unique combinations that allow you to find the idiosyncrasies the standardized programs won't know.

Without holistic planning, getting the numbers in the gym or miles on the road is only superficial. No training occurs in a bubble, so knowing what happened before a session is where the training stimulus actually comes from. A very common error is to set amateur athletes proud of their achievements in training, clocking the same numbers and miles as the elite yet unaware of the context. High numbers look impressive, yet it is the context that matters, and what the dilettante does once the top tier do weekly, and the sessions between, is what sets the overall rate of progress.

Recovery

You can only train as hard as you can recover. This is almost a law of training, but often escapes athletes who plot their preparation only by the average of their training sessions and overlook how they as athletes are developing.

The true indicator of progress is the *athlete*, not the training, and when vanguard objectives require long-term preparation, it is the athlete that must see the timeline through. This means said athletes' mental toughness must extend to more factors than just the time they spend training, which is something that may challenge how they currently think. Yes, it is important to have presence, control, patience, and focus during training, but maybe 10% of the overall time, what you do with all the other hours is where the difference really happens.

Elite athletes train and compete better, but they also rest, eat, sleep, recover, and play better too. Copying the gym or track sessions of top-tier athletes may feel like the right thing to be doing, but without understanding the rest, it is merely a shadow of what's actually going on. What matters most is the *ratio* of elite preparation, because this is what sets the volume of each element; how much is active time developing physical attributes, in ratio to time sleeping, relaxing, or in supportive recovery?

While novelty is not something to base active training on, it is very valuable as a protocol of recovery because it gives the athlete an alternative to the hard grind of incremental sport-specific preparation. Diversity in recovery methods and timelines both keeps life interesting and covers the most elements needed to really keep an athlete balanced.

Mental toughness relates to recovery in the discipline and creativity needed to recover properly, and the tougher the mind, the more effective the methods available. Whilst most of the recovery standards like diet, stretching, and manipulation have a great effect, mental toughness allows the athlete to go deeper into them in spite of an ego that may be pulling them in other directions.

The adept athlete understands when it is time to train and time to hold off–something surprisingly hard for the undeveloped athlete who is reliant only on schedules. Only when enough time and failure have accrued, can it be known what is the ideal timeline and how to allocate energy.

Effective recovery, just like effective training, means using a method until the required goal is achieved. Whilst it is normal for this to be well defined when pushing in the gym or on the field, few athletes consider recovery standards, let alone abide by them. A great advancement in recent years is access to decent quality heart rate monitors, that let anybody see trends in their daily condition. Whilst not always being very accurate, and needing other data to correlate, this is something that helps fill in the negative spaces around an athlete's scheduled training.

Eating

Diet is the obvious bedrock of all training, having its own huge body of knowledge beyond the scope of this book. Suffice it to say that without getting the basics right and eating to perform, no system of training will out-train bad eating. Overall, a proper diet is simple, but it's easy to be sucked into trivialities, minutiae, and scams thinking they are the shortcut to performance.

What matters most is having the mental toughness and creativity to bypass the cultural limits on which most eating is based on. Great athletic performance is seen across all cultures, meaning diets as diverse as Japanese to Ethiopian and Jamaican, are as supportive of performance as the latest supplements. Once basic requirements are met, the athlete must discern where novelty and identity take over, and those who are mentally tough will find more diversity to apply.

Eat according to your goals, which include all aspects of preparation, and enjoy what you eat so it avoids the beguiling nature of marketing and hype. The athlete that eats properly is fulfilling arguably the primary element of preparation and can train and recover better across the years needed to reach full potential.

Chapter 13: Detachment

A tough mind is a mind that can detach itself from the difficulties and rigors of athleticism, and perceive itself from a standpoint where the effort is in context. Detachment is often cited by endurance athletes as a factor in overcoming the effects of fatigue, stress, and pain. It is described as stepping away from the intensely intimate experience and seeing the performance from a perspective outside of yourself.

Indeed, at the most profound level, where experience is at its most extreme, detachment is the *only* way through for even the toughest of minds. All minds have a point where every attribute is exhausted, and the last course of action is to detach and play the game from another level.

This is not escapism nor ignorance, instead, it is letting go of the ego's hold on an experience. Nothing is being escaped from or ignored. Instead, all the effects of performance are still there, only they have been shifted in context to make them more manageable.

Yogic Disciplines

Disciplines like yoga and tai chi are ancient systems for learning to detach from the rigors of the body. Like in meditation, the mind is developed and controlled, in this case, to direct precise actions on the body, and in the process is seen to be a mechanism distinct from the body, like the driver is distinct from a car. Yoga-type disciplines are useful because the quiet and aware mindset allows the athlete to see deep into subtle reactions and see where the mind and body separate—or in some cases don't.

This highly refined interface is integral to mental toughness because it lets you see that so much of your behavior is simply a reaction to physical phenomena. Yoga, tai chi, etc., highlight this interface with movements and sequences that push reactions to the surface, making even the toughest mind acutely aware of how it is linked to the body.

Only through seeing this interplay can mental toughness really be developed, because it is here the athlete realizes how the ability to detach from the stress of the moment is key to keeping the mind level and focused. The mind that can go to extremes of physical stress and complexity yet keep itself aware and stable is a basic form of toughness, but can only be developed through precision and nuance over time.

Detachment usually means separating from the stress, pain, and limitations of the body that feedback to the mind and distracts it from clear thought. There are several stages to this process, and mostly they are manipulable, but it takes time and discipline to get the work done. Most athletes are aware of this, and the higher the skill level, usually the more an athlete includes practices similar to yoga or tai chi to work on them.

At this level, yoga, etc., need not include the esoteric or spiritual aspects that yoga and similar disciplines are often taught as part of. The separation has no effect on the attributes that apply to the athlete, and can be replaced with modern physiology or simply left out. There is no need for yoga or other systems that come from Eastern philosophical backgrounds to have any connection to unproven or religious elements, though it is worth the athlete's respect to look into what other cultures offer.

For the athlete, yoga to develop detachment and mental toughness must be more than just a minor compliment to other training, because it takes more than a peripheral amount of effort to see the benefits. Effective transfer to real-life performance—like with any effort—needs the accumulation of time, repetition, and effort, meaning more than an hour a week.

One of the advantages of yoga for mental toughness is that these disciplines have a lot of overlap with recovery and supplementary training such as warming up and cooling down, meaning that as they are learned, they can be incorporated into most aspects of preparation. Unlike the esoteric version, where yoga-type disciplines are a standalone practice, for the athlete, the principles apply to most other training.

At the physical level, yoga's well-known capacity for stretching and integrating movement and balance with breathing, things that have obvious connections to any athletic sport. Here the mind can get a deep and clear look into physical condition, including physical limitations around flexibility, balance and imbalance, range of motion, condition of the fascia, and posture.

Unlike nearly any other discipline, this degree of body awareness is developed rapidly because the athlete's mind is in a state of quietude, free of distraction, and the tempo of yoga or tai chi means weaknesses cannot be ignored. Unlike training focusing on speed, power, and endurance where a load of psychophysical feedback is high enough to override subtleties, things like tai chi expose them overtly.

This exposure to base-level physical weaknesses will be humbling and even alarming, confronting many of what mental toughness an athlete may think they possess. Like many of the other attributes we have discussed, these are the often overlooked or ignored aspects of mental toughness that some athletes do not recognize until it's too late.

Athletes who develop the basics of yoga, tai chi, or other such disciplines early, then apply them across their preparation, see big advantages. For many athletes, these are things they only become aware of later in their careers—often as a result of injury or deterioration of condition with age—almost always wishing they had known about it earlier.

The athlete who understands and uses these skills is less exposed to injury and has a greater capacity to mitigate it when it comes. The detachment learned is seen in an enhanced awareness of things affecting physical condition, an enhanced capacity to cope with and control pain, and because much of yoga, etc can be practiced in a low-effort state, this element of training can be continued whilst recovering.

Over time, and under the multiple annual cycles that almost all athletic sports have, yoga and tai chi retain consistency whatever the focus of the training phase. Obviously, this means continued long-term development, but it also contributes to mental toughness by becoming a regular indicator of mental and physical condition—something vital to the career of any serious athlete. Yoga gives a benchmark against which to assess things like heart rate, nerve recovery, mental state, muscular state, and structural imbalances, which is an insight into personal performance otherwise difficult to have.

Scale and Scope

It is easy to detach from a role by realizing the scale of the scenario, though this needs to be done with awareness and intent to avoid descending into fantasy. Done as a way to enhance performance and ability, recognizing the scale and scope of your efforts is fundamental to assessing where on the curve of ability you are, which lets you judge what you should be doing in order to progress.

Detachment lets the athlete view their sport and ability from outside their own singular perspective. In the context of the entire sport, or even the type of sport, detaching from your own tiny position and looking at where you fit in is something that is needed to determine how far you can go. Some sports do this within themselves, with rankings and competition results spanning the entire scene, with a good example being endurance running, with its point system that is globally open to any runner to join. This and similar systems have been central to these sports' recent development, pushing standards across a huge field to the benefit of everyone.

Scale refers to how much is involved in your sport, meaning the number of people and events going on. For some sports with huge communities and literally millions of participants, making it to the elite levels means a massive and complicated process. The scale of an athlete's efforts will be determined by many things, with mental toughness being central to it all because this is what lets them perform at a competitive level across the time needed to prevail. Every year, dozens of athletes see excellent results that show a spike on the scale, but only those mentally tough enough will sustain the performance to rise to an elite level.

The athlete who is detached enough to see their position in the grand scheme of things can judge where they need to perform to move upwards in their field. It is rarely enough to simply excel at a local, isolated level–most outliers or freak talents are the stuff of fantasy–and most athletes need to get beyond their niche so they can take their performance higher.

Scope means what you can do and how you can apply your abilities, and mental toughness is an obvious central factor in this, because it can be a shock to realize what high-level performance demands. Without pushing the scope of your ability, you cannot rise above your current performance, so it is important to see what others are doing and allow their influence to inform you. This means detaching from the current views, which may be the products of a lifetime, and allowing new ideas that will change how you perform. This is a common thing to see in sports like mixed martial arts and endurance athletics, where athletes regularly seek new methods to increase the scope of their skills. It is no coincidence that these same sports are synonymous with mental toughness, with this correlation being a prime indicator of an athlete's future performance.

Scale and scope, as the athlete progresses, become increasingly central to preparation as performance gets better. First, the athlete breaks beyond what the local scope and scale of ability offer, pushing up to a wider level where they are set against other athletes from a bigger pool of ability. This progress through levels is always confronting at each stage, exposing the athlete to higher ability and more commitment that requires a tougher and more adaptable mind.

In rare cases, the athlete will stop, in most cases because they have reached the pinnacle of their sport, but in most cases, because their mental toughness has met its threshold. This is the stark reality of athletic performance, and even the most talented and gifted athletes will be ultimately limited by what their minds can tolerate. The simple cold fact is those with the most mental toughness go further because they can stand back from themselves, see where they are in the field, and have the wherewithal and attributes to take things further.

Chapter 14: Stillness

It is the scope of the mind that determines how tough it is, with your degree of mental toughness being how far your mind can go before it starts feeling the effects of overextension. Mental toughness accepts a huge amount of stress and intensity, but only as much as the other extremity of stillness and centeredness can anchor.

Mental toughness does not mean working at the extremities of your character all the time. Athletes can indeed maintain a peak level of performance for weeks or even months, but the intensity at some point will give out unless you have a mental space of stillness to phase through to keep everything in check.

Constant competition, focus, and intensity make the mind restless and hyper-alert which can affect decisiveness and the ability to relax and will eventually corrode the mind rather than toughen it. To avoid this and keep the faculties sharp, this state of stillness is where the mind can decompress and return to the center in a state far from its competitive edge.

Stillness is not something that will develop without intention, and like patience, it is an attribute around which other faculties function better because the traffic in your mind is given a way to decongest. Like meditation, stillness is cultivated by intentionally finding and expanding the aspects of your character where your mind finds itself content with no need for reaction. This is found by regularly stepping back from the leading edge of your mind, suspending the constant need for reaction, and letting the mind settle, so the feedback loop of attention eases.

The Center of the Cyclone

Stillness is the true test of mental toughness because beyond performing better and being more tenacious it is the capacity to remain calm and still whilst all around you is caught up in the heat of competition that sets the really tough mindset apart. At this level, toughness doesn't pertain to withstanding the bombardment of pressure, instead, it is about maintaining balance and structure to keep the athlete's mind strong against forces pulling it outwards.

Beyond the casual level, athleticism becomes increasingly complex, stressful, distracting, and invasive, and without the capacity to find stillness to retreat to, the competition becomes not for other athletes but to prevail over burnout. This is an often-unmentioned element of elite performance but is usually the factor that limits how far an athlete can go. They may train better, be smarter, more creative, and more motivated—but without a state of stillness to center in, the energy equation just can't balance out.

Like the center of an actual cyclone, here the imperative is to anchor the self to faculties that give the athlete clarity and awareness of the entire dynamic scenario of performance but not be sucked out into it. It is easy to be drawn into the drama and ego of competition, and only the strongest of minds can keep still and free of compulsion as competition soars.

Where this matters most is in the spotlight of performance, where the influence of other competitors and spectators is most intense. This is when athletes can become overwhelmed by the pressure from outside themselves, and make corrupted decisions that in an instant change how things will play out.

This is the very nature of competition and the true test of the toughened mind. Even the most developed of minds will find here the things they did and didn't get right. Like the cyclone, to lose equilibrium here means being pulled out into the complexity and confusion of competition, which is what separates the best from those still needing more development. Many top athletes talk about this scenario, almost all of them using analogies like cyclones or storms, as well as the conclusion that it is mental toughness that prevails.

This centered state of stillness can only be developed by applying the intent and detachment that come with the many aspects of mental toughness. As we have progressed through the many various attributes, the capacity for toughness has risen, and it is here at the hypocenter of performance that it stops being about external pressure and starts being about it from within. All the other factors in mental toughness, like detachment, self-validation, control, and focus, culminate here to give the mind an incredible degree of internal strength.

Outside of the intensity of competition, this state of stillness, is immune to the restlessness that can plague an athlete yet to develop mental toughness to this degree. Stillness lets the mind wander and explore, but unlike restlessness, which is searching for novelty, with a center to return to, the toughened mind can travel far but still return. Indeed, by developing a centered, still, mind, the athlete moves beyond many of the trivial and inconsequential things that trap the untrained mind into a constant battle with boredom, perhaps being the most important attribute of mental toughness.

Consciousness

There is the profoundly philosophical aspect to consciousness, the existentialist matter of what it is to be aware in a world that boils down to seemingly unconscious elements, and there is the practical aspect of being aware and engaged in the things you do. Whilst many athletes have, of course, also expounded on the former, it is this everyday awareness where mental toughness is most felt.

This is where athleticism becomes not an end in itself, but a means to the end of what athleticism can bring. This was something the ancient Greeks thought about, with the original

Olympics to demonstrate how athleticism was the embodiment of their philosophy of life, and is something the Chinese have pursued in martial arts as the expression of Daoist principles.

Now, it is easy to get lost in the esoterica of all this, but it is also well known that at the peak of performance, these questions and thoughts often arise. The baseball coach who develops a philosophy for the team, the gymnast who seeks the ultimate expression of strength, the marathon runner who is chasing the limit of human potential, and the Bluewater yachtsman who pits himself against global weather systems on the edge of extreme risk—these are things that summon elements of character outside of what normal athleticism is about.

The athlete who touches this part of their character is looking into what it means to compete and where performance can go, which are the things that define the very sports that they do. This is where real changes in the direction of athleticism can be felt, but it takes mental toughness to pursue these ideas to see actual results.

Yes, we are all conscious of taking on sport at some level, with 99.9% of us happy to just play the game as it is, as a part of life that expresses our ideas about physical competition, pride in our performance, and a chance to excel at something with clearly defined rules. But some athletes, given the opportunity to see what their characters really are made of, will find sport as the thing that shows them more of life. Beyond the physical training and the psychological pursuit of better performance, in the stillness that comes with focus, identity, and detachment, the ideas will be about bigger things.

Mental toughness is the only faculty of mind that will get an athlete both into and through this level of thinking. It takes the combined elements of the many things that lead to it for the mind to think this way, and those same elements to be strong and cohesive enough to reflect on the role athletic performance plays in their lives.

Some athletes will find all this makes them better people, and more able to express their ideas in a diverse and evolving world. For them being a good athlete is about more than the speed, strength, power, precision, endurance, and other qualities just to hit a ball or move the distance; and is about a way of thinking that has applications in other things.

In its way, this is pure athleticism, where the goal of performance and winning is not to beat others but to beat the limitations of the self. This is where the athlete's career is not seen as culminating in their peak performance on the field, but as what it has made them compared to what they would have been otherwise.

Chapter 15: Gratitude

Never forget what mental toughness is *for*. This can sound like an oblique thing, but despite everything that goes into it, mental toughness itself is not the objective, and losing sight of that can result in losing the best things in life.

Dig away at mental toughness, and it becomes apparent what it means to be as effective as you can be, and not just as an athlete but as a person. Real progress is only made with a complete perspective to act on, and the lessons of athleticism flow through all of life. What this means is that your performance is the result of a whole body of knowledge, and all of it has come from those who went before. The sports we pursue, the standards we use, and the goals that are set—all the way down to the shoes that we wear and the gravel that we stand on—have come from the ideas and efforts of others.

By choosing to be athletes, we have chosen to be part of traditions and histories that have stood the test of time. In some cases, those histories have long and significant ramifications, containing elements of society as it changed. In other cases, the history of a sport is still in the making, with potential only being realized and the future exciting and close, making the athlete integral, if only to bring momentum in numbers.

These are all things that deserve our gratitude, not in some sycophantic way, but simply because if it is worth our energy, it is worth acknowledging the energy of others who had similar ideas. This is not to put others on some sort of pedestal, but to realize we are part of communities that can maintain the ideas and standards that keep people together in the pursuit of human performance.

Showing Respect

Real respect is not shown with words or gestures, it is shown by what you do with those things. We can all say the right words, shake the right hands, and post the right things on social media, but to those who choose to look, real respect comes in other forms.

Respect is showing the value you place on something or someone, and only really happens when you do that thing yourself. Of course, you can *like* anything you choose, but until you like it enough to act on it, it does not become respect.

As an athlete, the way to show respect for an idea or person is to put that thing into action. If a top sprinter has your admiration, show your respect for their abilities by adopting the aspects of them that matter to you. This doesn't necessarily mean copying what another athlete does—something that needs a large body of other information besides simple respect to make effective—but it does mean learning and applying the methods of greater athletes as contributions to the sport and taking them up to be part of pushing the sport forward.

It is important to show respect for those you admire and the things that they achieve because this is how the methodologies of athletic sports evolve. The goal here is not some kind of cult of personality by only respecting the person, but to recognize them as the protagonist of their actions that are part of raising standards for everyone.

Respect can be shown by recognizing the process and contributions of other athletes any time the effects of their contributions are felt. In some sports, this is as easy as mentioning names associated with styles or techniques, and in other sports, it can mean acknowledging them in reports and interviews. What matters most here is to show your performance in the light of others who have influenced it, to show that these sports are evolving and progressing over time.

Beyond the sport itself, it is important to recognize and respect other factors that have made contributions to your performance, from other people who have helped to respect the environment and fairness of the game. No sport happens in isolation, being always the product of the place and time where they occur, and showing you acknowledge and understand that relationship is part of demonstrating that you know the gravity of your efforts.

Respect at this level is not only about admiration and accolades, it is about understanding your position in a much larger process than simply hitting a ball or running around a track. All competition is the meeting of individuals who come from a diversity of backgrounds, and at the highest root of athleticism as expounded by the Greek philosophers, this is what is really what is being demonstrated.

In the pursuit of your sporting ideals, it takes innumerable factors and elements along the way to make it all happen, and just as it is good practice to acknowledge the efforts of those who contributed to putting food on the table, it is good practice to recognize what contributes to you competing. There need be nothing religious or even spiritual in this because there are more than enough tangible and undisputed factors to count. By simply showing respect for what you are doing you show that you understand the place of it all in a world where not everything is guaranteed.

Perhaps the best example of this respect is found in martial arts, where every school and style has the tradition of recognizing the chain of teachers and methods that came together to result in what exists now. Martial arts being what they are, these methods have been tried and tested in the reality of competition, so what has made it down through time is the product of people who cared and put themselves on the line. Members of these sports are judged by their sincerity, where the very space they are in is given the respect of a place away from the corruption and tenuous honesty of the outside world. This place is reserved for the pursuit of excellence, and respect is what holds that together, and showing sincere acknowledgment of that is the price of entry.

Grace Under Pressure

Athleticism is one of the few *proven* things that can turn even the most corrupted life around, and for that, it deserves respect simply because it works. Not all claimed methods for advancing the human condition are either effective or real, but the value of progressing as an athlete almost always improves character. A common saying among the military is that athletic ability is the *only* true measure of a person because it is the only thing that cannot be bought, taken, faked, stolen, or mimicked—what the athlete attains is exactly the outcome of their efforts, that is the distillation of everything about them and by which they are judged in the real world of performance.

Without respect and gratitude, athleticism is little more than a game, because of the things that are competed for becoming trivial and selfish. When gratitude and respect are absent performance becomes corruptible, and about things other than the process of betterment and excellence. We see this on occasions when athletes are caught doping, cheating, or using unfair means—things that are not illegal but that lower the standards of the sport. From drugs in cycling to bottled oxygen on Mt Everest, when the standard is not set by the leading edge, the whole field is corrupted, and achievement stagnates as it is overtaken by those opting for the easiest option.

Anyone can be grateful when things are going well, and to only see yourself in the light of your successes is a sign of a shallow and untested mind. Mountaineers have a paradigm where they judge each other not by what they have summited but by what has turned them around, because in standards of that sport—where risk is very real—it is their ability to stay alive and return that is their true measure.

Those sorts of sports are easy to find gratitude within, the risks to life obviously being very humbling, but all sports have their angles where gratitude will be found, and the athlete is measured in ways other than performance. This is the ultimate role of mental toughness within athleticism—to push not just the athlete, but the sport itself into higher levels of dynamism.

An informed review of the past decade in any sport will show how performance is evolving and the directions being taken. In a world devoted to convenience and comfort, the many fields of athleticism are some of the few that run counter to this, concerned instead with pushing into ever more difficult realms. Speeds are getting faster, distances are getting longer, ability pushed higher, and the very environments some sports take place in are being pushed towards greater extremes. This demonstrates a deep human will to prevail, with the capacity to overcome as a fundamental trait.

Conclusion

All things being equal, the bottom line is that mental toughness is what decides those who prevail. We have shown here that this mindset of being toughened mentally is a many-faceted thing, but as a whole, the combination of these elements is greater than the sum of the parts.

Mental toughness is the single attribute that brings all other attributes together, both as the connecting factor in every aspect of the athlete's character and as the defining character trait when it comes time to perform. Consistent and consolidated development of mental toughness is what builds the athlete that can take the competition to the highest level, where they not only prevail at their sport but can potentially influence the sport itself. This is where athleticism goes from being just a psycho-physical pursuit and touches on what it means to excel in a world most often choose to just sit and watch.

Perhaps most importantly it is mental toughness that makes the athlete prevail over themselves, to rise above where they come from and the rules of the game. This may be as simple as scoring better in a sport based on points, as integral as finishing in an event based on endurance, or as definitive as setting records or survival in something where everything is on the line.

The Difference

Develop these traits and the difference will be seen in everyday life but will be most noticeable when it comes to performance. These days athletic performance, in general, is so high due to the mass availability of elite-level information, it is the single-digit percentiles that make the difference, and it is here that mental toughness matters most.

Prevailing as an athlete rapidly becomes about much more than the competition or even the game. And becomes about the self and how far you will go to succeed. This is exactly the place where mental toughness makes the difference, by raising the bar of what you can achieve. The mentally tougher athlete trains harder, trains more, trains smarter, and prepares more efficiently even before performance begins, and it is these very elements that relate more to results than any other. By the time performance comes around the majority of what mental toughness brings to the athlete is well in motion, to be finally thrown into the ring where the clarity and confidence mental toughness brings sees the athlete through. Without the base they have developed nothing makes much difference at the sharp end of the performance, and it is here that the mentally tough athletes is obviously better.

Watch any elite-level performance, and you are seeing mental toughness in action. For whatever genetics, fortune, and talent is present it is mental toughness that got them ahead of all the others with the same advantages.

The mentally tough athlete has higher thresholds for nearly every vector that imposes limitations, like pain, fatigue, attention to detail, recovery, confidence, and many others. These things have all been trained in the lead-up to the big day whether it's a game series, a race, an event, or an expedition, and it all comes together in that final display.

You will see the difference between athletes with greater toughness as they will be less affected by the excitement of performance and ability to make critical decisions with greater confidence because their bar for chaos and extreme application of ability is higher. This may simply be the outcome of having trained for more years, been through failures, or having better preparation, and it will be their mindset that allows tougher decisions that will see how far their performance can go.

Stay Strong
Stay Consistent
Stay Healthy
&
Keep Developing Yourself

Level Up

Thank You

Thank you for taking the time to read this book on mental toughness. If you found it valuable and it resonated with you, I kindly request that you consider leaving an honest review. Your feedback is greatly appreciated and can help others make informed decisions about reading this book.

References

Beck, N. M. (2012, May). *Mental toughness: An analysis of sex, race, and mood.* ProQuest. https://proquest.com/openview/60b49e0db636 c159fa1b8310b8feb8d0/1?pq-origsite=gscholar&cbl=18750

Brace, A. W., George, K., & Lovell, G. P. (2020). Mental toughness and self-efficacy of elite ultra-marathon runners. *PLOS ONE*, 15(11), e0241284. https://doi.org/10.1371/journal.pone.0241284

Caddick, N., & Ryall, E. (2012). The Social Construction of "Mental Toughness" – a Fascistoid Ideology? *Journal of the Philosophy of Sport*, 39(1), 137–154. https://doi.org/10.1080/00948705.2012.67506 8

Connaughton, D., Hanton, S., & Jones, G. (2010). The Development and Maintenance of Mental Toughness in the World's Best Performers. *The Sport Psychologist*, 24(2), 168–193. https://doi.org/10.1123/tsp.24.2.168

Connaughton, D., Wadey, R., Hanton, S., & Jones, G. (2008). The development and maintenance of mental toughness: Perceptions of elite performers. *Journal of Sports Sciences*, 26(1), 83–95. https://doi.org/10.1080/02640410701310958

Cowden, R. G., Joynt, S., Crust, L., Hook, J. N., & Worthington, E. L. (2018). *How do mentally tough athletes overcome self-directed anger, shame, and criticism? A self-forgiveness mediation analysis.* Repository.nwu.ac.za. http://repository.nwu.ac.za/handle/10394/31721

Crust, L. (2007). Mental toughness in sport: A review. *International Journal of Sport and Exercise Psychology*, 5(3), 270–290. https://doi.org/10.1080/1612197x.2007.9671836

Crust, L. (2009). The relationship between mental toughness and affect intensity. *Personality and Individual Differences*, 47(8), 959–963. https://doi.org/10.1016/j.paid.2009.07.023

Crust, L., & Azadi, K. (2010). Mental toughness and athletes' use of psychological strategies. *European Journal of Sport Science*, 10(1), 43–51. https://doi.org/10.1080/17461390903049972

Crust, L., & Keegan, R. (2010). Mental toughness and attitudes to risk-taking. *Personality and Individual Differences*, 49(3), 164–168. https://doi.org/10.1016/j.paid.2010.03.026

Drees, M. J., & Mack, M. G. (2012, December). *An Examination of Mental Toughness over the Course of a Competitive Season.* ProQuest. https://proquest.com/openview/2799d524d62d576da79d6aff4cca1633/1?pq-origsite=gscholar&cbl=30153

Gucciardi, D. F., Gordon, S., & Dimmock, J. A. (2009). Advancing mental toughness research and theory using personal construct psychology. *International Review of Sport and Exercise Psychology*, 2(1), 54–72. https://doi.org/10.1080/17509840802705938

Gucciardi, D. F., Hanton, S., Gordon, S., Mallett, C. J., & Temby, P. (2015). The Concept of Mental Toughness: Tests of Dimensionality, Nomological Network, and Traitness. *Journal of Personality*, 83(1), 26–44. https://doi.org/10.1111/jopy.12079

Jackman, P. C., Crust, L., & Swann, C. (2017). *Further examining the relationship between mental toughness and dispositional flow in sport.* A mediation analysis | IJSP Online. http://www.ijsp-online.com/abstract/view/48/356

Jackman, P. C., Swann, C., & Crust, L. (2016). Exploring athletes' perceptions of the relationship between mental toughness and dispositional flow in sport. *Psychology of Sport and Exercise*, 27(27), 56–65. https://doi.org/10.1016/j.psychsport.2016.07.007

Jones, G., Hanton, S., & Connaughton, D. (2007). A Framework of Mental Toughness in the World's Best Performers. *The Sport Psychologist*, 21(2), 243–264. https://doi.org/10.1123/tsp.21.2.243

Jones, M. I., & Parker, J. K. (2018). Mindfulness mediates the relationship between mental toughness and pain catastrophizing in cyclists. *European Journal of Sport Science*, 18(6), 872–881.

https://doi.org/10.1080/17461391.2018.147845
0

julianservice23. (2021a, February 25). *Powerful ways to Develop Mental Toughness.* MINDSET. https://high3rmindset.com/post/develop-mental-toughness

julianservice23. (2021b, May 20). *Mental Toughness Training for Athletes.* MINDSET. https://high3rmindset.com/post/mental-toughness-training-for-athletes

julianservice23. (2021c, June 17). *Mental Conditioning Training: Why this is a KEY part of mental toughness.* MINDSET. https://high3rmindset.com/post/mental-conditioning-training-why-this-is-a-key-part-of-mental-toughness

Kuan, G., & Roy, J. (2007). Goal Profiles, Mental Toughness and its Influence on Performance Outcomes among Wushu Athletes. *Journal of Sports Science & Medicine*, 6(CSSI-2), 28–33. https://ncbi.nlm.nih.gov/pmc/articles/PMC380 9050/

Kudlackova, K. (2011). *Electronic Theses, Treatises and Dissertations The Graduate School.* Diginole.lib.fsu.edu. https://diginole.lib.fsu.edu/islandora/object/fsu :181168/datastream/PDF/view

Lin, Y., Mutz, J., Clough, P. J., & Papageorgiou, K. A. (2017). Mental Toughness and Individual Differences in Learning, Educational and Work Performance, Psychological Well-being, and

Personality: *A Systematic Review. Frontiers in Psychology,* 8. https://doi.org/10.3389/fpsyg.2017.01345

Lohan, A. (2021). Athletes' performance with yoga and associated exercises. *ACADEMICIA: An International Multidisciplinary Research Journal,* 11(9), 408–414. https://doi.org/10.5958/2249-7137.2021.01931.5

Madrigal, L. (2017, March). *Gender and the Relationships Among Mental Toughness, Hardiness, Optimism and Coping in Collegiate Athletics: A Structural Equation Modeling Approach.* ProQuest. https://proquest.com/openview/6843b6babaf7f 1ee3bce8064cbecc77e/1?pq-origsite=gscholar&cbl=30153

Nicholls, A. R., Polman, R. C. J., Levy, A. R., & Backhouse, S. H. (2008). Mental toughness, optimism, pessimism, and coping among athletes. *Personality and Individual Differences,* 44(5), 1182–1192. https://doi.org/10.1016/j.paid.2007.11.011

Sheard, M. (2012). *Mental Toughness.* Routledge. https://doi.org/10.4324/9780203103548

Sorensen, S., Jarden, A., & Schofield, G. (2016). Lay perceptions of mental toughness: Understanding conceptual similarities and differences between lay and sporting contexts. *International Journal of Wellbeing,* 6(3), 71–95. https://doi.org/10.5502/ijw.v6i3.551

About the Author

HIGH3R MINDSET was founded in 2020 by Julian Service who played NCAA and Pro level baseball for many years. Due to his passion for health, fitness and just helping others, he felt there was the overwhelming need for a mental health advocacy and mental strength guidance. Through years of trial and error, plus mentoring of ones with more experience to share, we have attained an understanding of fitness and health at a significantly deeper level. Mental and physical health affects everyone, regardless of rich or poor, and especially in the current times we are living in. Therefore, we chose to broaden our horizons, and reach out to as many people as possible to provide our knowledge.

www.high3rmindset.com